I Felt a Right One

… and now I feel a right one again

Karen Tighe

Copyright © 2013 Karen Tighe

The moral right of the author has been asserted.

Apart from any fair dealing for the purposes of research or private study, or criticism or review, as permitted under the Copyright, Designs and Patents Act 1988, this publication may only be reproduced, stored or transmitted, in any form or by any means, with the prior permission in writing of the publishers, or in the case of reprographic reproduction in accordance with the terms of licences issued by the Copyright Licensing Agency. Enquiries concerning reproduction outside those terms should be sent to the publishers.

Matador
9 Priory Business Park,
Wistow Road, Kibworth Beauchamp,
Leicestershire. LE8 0RX
Tel: (+44) 116 279 2299
Fax: (+44) 116 279 2277
Email: books@troubador.co.uk
Web: www.troubador.co.uk/matador

ISBN 978 1780884 639

British Library Cataloguing in Publication Data.
A catalogue record for this book is available from the British Library.

Printed and bound in the UK by TJ International, Padstow, Cornwall
Typeset in 11pt Aldine401 BT Roman by Troubador Publishing Ltd, Leicester, UK

Matador is an imprint of Troubador Publishing Ltd

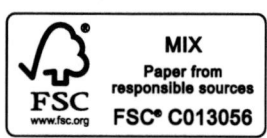

No reader could fail to be moved by her strong and positive approach to every woman's nightmare – the diagnosis of cancer in the breast. Her account of how she, with the support of her husband, family and friends, tackled the difficult months that followed is moving – and uplifting. She is clearly a person with great grit and determination.

Vivienne Shuster – Publishing agent

I read the first seven chapters (as I feared – impossible to put down!) and I think this is a brilliant book; such a good, uplifting story with a real insight on the cancer journey. I want to make an order immediately as I would like to be able to give it to newly diagnosed cancer patients in my surgery.

Dr Colleen Wood

The book is a wonderful manifestation of your own energy and personality, perhaps the greatest asset of all when faced with such a difficult diagnosis. I greatly enjoyed the style and enthusiasm. It is always interesting to see the journey from a patient's perspective and, I suspect, your words would give enormous comfort and encouragements to others embarking on a similar trip.

Adam Searle – BDS MB BS FRCS FRCS(Plast)

A very easy and refreshing story and one that will resonate with many. Those who know you will laugh out loud a lot and imagine you very vividly, those who don't will be inspired by your courage and your attitude, and many will identify with your emotions which are so vividly documented.

Lisa Allera

*To John, Lizzie and Marcus,
for their love and inspiration.*

All profits from the publication of this book will be given equally to two charities: Breast Cancer Care and St Luke's Hospice.

Contents

Introduction	ix
Discovery	1
Let's Get Checked	4
The Tests	10
The Results	14
Start Spreading the News	17
So What's the Treatment?	25
The Calm Before the Storm	29
The Operation	32
Recuperation	41
Chemotherapy – Poison that Makes You Better	54
Letting My Hair Down or Rather Out!	61
Just When You Think it is All Going So Well	72
A Light at the End of the Tunnel Gets Darker Before Getting lighter Again	87
A Life Changing Experience	93
The End of the Poison and Time to Get Nuked!	97

I FELT A RIGHT ONE...

A Girl's Got to Do What a Girl's Got to Do	105
The Treatment Comes to an End	109
Getting Back to Normal and the Waiting Game	113
A Smashing Time!	121
Planning	126
They Can Rebuild You, they Have the Technology	134
I Can Feel a Right one Again	145
Committing Pen to Paper	157
It's Only Pain	160
A Few Minor Adjustments Including the Dog Ears	163
No You Don't Have Bone Cancer, You Just Need a Hip Replacement	175
We Can Rebuild You Phase II	186
Travel Broadens the Mind and Brings Friends Closer	193
Coming of Age	202
A New Nipple and a Proper Tattoo	204
Life is a Journey	210
Acknowledgements	214

Introduction

I get the impression that many people would like to write a book, but never try.

I can honestly say that I really never did want to write a book, partly because I didn't think anyone would want to read anything I felt like writing and also I didn't think I wrote very well. Years spent working on corporate communications in the mobile phone industry meant that I can write really good, boring stuff!

However, when life throws you a curved ball and you get cancer, you really start to think about things in a different way. Why not write a book? Now I had something to say that people might be interested to read, so why not try.

My motivation came from lots of friends who said that they liked reading the update emails sent to them during my treatment and that I should write a book. I had been writing a kind of diary, in the hope that getting my thoughts on paper would actually help me sort out how I felt about being ill, so I had some material to work with.

Anyway, with much encouragement and determination I have decided to write this book, even if it doesn't get published, just for the hell of it. It will be an accomplishment. Something I can say that I have done.

It may help before you start reading to understand a little about me. I am now fifty years old, married to John with two children,

I FELT A RIGHT ONE...

Lizzie and Marcus. I had a career in marketing and then retrained to be a primary school teacher in 2005. I am horribly organised, which drives most people mad and I am incredibly positive. I am either living my life at 100mph or I am comatose, with little variance in between. It is really only my family that get to see me comatose, so most people think I never stop. Duracell bunny-esque!

Organising things, being involved and just generally being active is how I live my life. I am very extrovert and generally wear my heart on my sleeve. If I am happy you'll know it, if I am cross you'll know it. But most importantly I always try to see the good in things. Sometimes that is really hard, but once you get practiced at it (which I am) the silver linings in even the largest cloud will soon become evident.

I like to treat other people as I would like to be treated myself in fact; now I am working on treating them like I think they might want to be treated, for as you know, we are all different.

Finally, if I can write a book that people actually want to buy, then I can raise money for two amazing charities. Breast Cancer Care and St Luke's Hospice – both near to my heart. One almost literally and one metaphorically.

Karen Tighe

CHAPTER 1

Discovery

So what do you do when you find that your nipple is no longer on straight?

This is what I am thinking whilst on holiday. It is the summer of 2008 and the Tighe family depart for the US on a three week holiday. Lizzie is thirteen and Marcus eleven; good ages to manage the long flights and the amount of moving around we have planned. We are starting in Florida to have a week hitting the theme parks. We all really like stomach churning rides – the bigger and twistier the better. Then we are going to go to Kansas City, to stay with a friend that John used to work with at Kodak and her family, then to New York for a few days. John is then going to come home and I am going to take the children to North Carolina to stay with a friend from university – a really exciting trip where we will get both the chance to be foot-weary tourists, but also to relax in the company of good friends.

So we are right at the beginning of our trip, staying at our timeshare in Florida; the first time we have stayed in the resort since we bought it fifteen years before. I am lying in the very large and luxurious whirlpool bath, wallowing like a hippo. In fact I am thinking that I am becoming a little too much like a hippo. It feels very decadent, but after a long day at Disney, your feet and legs ache so much and a warm bath just hits the spot. The way I look at it is, if you are going to spend all that money then you need to make the most of it, so a bath to ensure you are fully fit for another full day on your feet is actually an investment more than a luxury!

Whilst lying soaking, I hear the sound of the Beijing Olympics which is on the TV in the lounge. We have been watching it most evenings, laughing at the unsurprisingly hugely biased coverage given by the US television stations. I lay back and take a look at my bigger-than-I-would-really-like body and focus on my chest.

Now my chest is not difficult to miss. It is hard to believe that as a child, my brothers called me 'currents on a blackboard'. I was a late developer, but once I started I didn't seem to stop. One friend always used to greet me with "How are the both of you!" Two children and gaining some weight had just made them even bigger. So my large G cup breasts are not difficult to miss, even with my poor eyesight and without my glasses.

What I see makes me sit up straight. To me, it looks like my right nipple is not on straight. I put my glasses on and have a really good look, then start to gently feel my whole right breast. I feel the left one for good measure and can definitely detect a lump in the right one. I am not too worried as I have always had lumpy breasts. I have had lumps before and they have always just been lumps. These were cysts, which I had had aspirated – where the doctor puts a needle into the lump and drains off the fluid – an interesting if slightly weird experience. In fact, as a large chested lady I have often hoped that aspiration may make the breast slightly smaller, but to no avail!

Later that evening, when John comes to bed and I am getting undressed, I ask him to have a look at my chest. I ask if to him it looks lopsided or different in any way. He carefully looks, enjoys having a feel to check them out, but does confirm that he can feel a lump too. John is also quite relaxed about it as he has seen me experience several mammograms and aspirations before. We talk about it and say it is probably just a lump and I'll get it checked out when I get home to the UK.

At the end of the holiday, when I am staying with my physioterrorist (sorry physiotherapist) friend Karen, I mention the lump to her. Karen is sympathetic and gently reminds me to make sure that I go to the doctor to get it checked when I get home. She mentions that if I were to have tests then I should ensure that I get an 'enhanced MRI' as this best shows any problems. She is quite careful, it seems to me, not to say the word cancer. I log the MRI information in my memory banks, which are definitely not as reliable as they used to be, and get on with the last few days of the holiday.

Although I am being nonchalant about all this, I do have to admit that I am, at this stage, a little worried about this lump. This one is different to any I have had before. Certainly no lump I had before had changed the shape of my breast or nipple in any way, so in my mind the thought that it is breast cancer creeps in, only to be shoved to the back, as there is nothing I can do until I get home.

CHAPTER 2

Let's Get Checked

We fly back into Heathrow on Friday at lunchtime. John picks us up from the airport and the children go straight off to scout camp. I clear all the washing and go straight back to work on the Monday.

I retrained to be a teacher in 2005 and have been working part-time since then. However, I am now going back to work full-time and am really excited to have a class all to myself. I have been given the same year group as I had last year (as a two day a week part-timer). We have two training days and then the children come back on the Wednesday.

I call the GP during that week and make an appointment for Monday 8th September. I also have a really sore neck and am having trouble swallowing without pain, so in reality I am more worried about this than I am about the lump in my breast.

The following Monday I go to my doctor's surgery and see Dr Perreira, a lovely young GP with an excellent manner. She makes a referral to a consultant, Michael Burke, who I have seen two or three times before. I am able to ask for a private referral, as when John started a new job only six months ago he got private medical insurance for the whole family. The delightful Dr Perreria is not too concerned about the lumps or the sore throat, but is sympathetic, supportive and generally very kind. She has a very gentle manner and never seems to rush you, even though you may have gone over your allotted time.

I call the Clementine Churchill Hospital and cannot get an appointment to see Mr Burke for two and a half weeks – towards the end of September. Again, I am not too worried and am happy to wait to see someone who I already know and who has treated me before, so I just get on with my work.

Now, at this time, John's new job takes him all over Europe. In fact he is out of the country about three weeks out of four. He leaves early on a Monday and gets back on a Friday. Both the children and I miss him, but he is really enjoying the challenge of this job. On the night that I have my appointment to see the consultant, John is in Spain, so I go on my own.

Sitting in the large waiting area at the hospital, I start thinking, really for the first time, about the process and the possible outcomes of this appointment. I am going to have to show my chest off to a strange man, not for the first time and so I am not too worried about this. Will I have to have tests? I hope it just needs aspirating and that will be that. A few minutes later, out walks the consultant, who shakes me warmly by the hand and takes me into his consulting room.

I explain what I have found and the consultant asks me to sit on the bed, strip to the waist and prepare for the examination. He asks questions, prods, pokes, palpates and then gets me to lie down. He puts some cold jelly (why is it never warm!) on the breast and then proceeds to perform an ultrasound examination. As soon as he is finished he gives me some tissue to clean myself up with and tells me to get dressed and come and sit down. Whilst all this is going on, I am talking to him about people we both know, medical staff working for St Luke's Hospice.

As soon as he says to me to clean myself up, I know that there is something wrong. Normally the consultant chats through the ultrasound and says that there is nothing to worry about. Although it is several years since I have seen him, I remember the drill.

I FELT A RIGHT ONE...

The consultant says he thinks there is an abnormality in the breast that needs to be investigated further. He says that I need to have a mammogram and a biopsy and he would like it done this Saturday. I go into autopilot and ask what his concerns are. He comments that he can feel a noticeable difference in the breast and that the change in shape is indicative of several possibilities. He goes on to say that the only way to determine what the problem is will be to have the tests. He asks me to make another appointment for the following Wednesday, when the results of the tests will be available. I thank him in a daze and walk out.

So now my mind starts to race. I have had a couple of mammograms before and I am not worried on that score, apart from having my chest squeezed as thin as a pancake! It is the word 'biopsy' that is so scary. This is the test which determines whether the lump that you have been trying to pretend is just the same as all the others, is actually cancer or not. I walk round to the imaging department and make an appointment for that Saturday at midday.

I get in the car and call John, but it goes through to voicemail. I need to talk to someone so call my sister-in-law Zoe. Well, she is not really my sister-in-law, she is John's identical twin brother's wife (let's call her sister-in-law, it is a lot easier!). Eammon, John's twin, says she is out. I say it is not urgent as I don't want to worry him and he says he'll get Zoe to call me later.

Now I really need to talk to someone and so I call Sarah. Sarah is a good friend and her son, Thomas, has been in the same class as my daughter Lizzie since reception. Sarah is a nurse and to my great relief answers.

I tell her what has happened and burst into tears. Sarah offers to come round, but I say not to worry and that I am just overreacting. It is really because I can't talk to John that I am upset. I also do not want to worry the children just yet; if Sarah comes round and I am crying, it would get them upset. There may yet be nothing to be upset about, so I go inside and act completely normally with the children. John calls back later and I tell him what has happened. He feels helpless so far away, but is suitably sympathetic and makes all the right noises, tells me not to worry and that it still may be nothing.

The next morning at about 7.45am I am in my classroom marking books, when Chris, the head teacher, walks in to tell me something. When he has told me, he asks if I am alright and I say that I am OK. Chris is perceptive and probes a little deeper and I burst out with the fact that I found out last night that I have to have a breast tissue biopsy on Saturday. I apologise for the outburst and explain that I am sure it's nothing.

Every time I say this to someone I know it is a lie. I know in my heart of hearts that I have cancer and it is just a matter of time until it is confirmed. I know that I shouldn't think negatively about it and that thinking it will happen will only make it happen. Equally, I don't want to be an ostrich, pretending that nothing is wrong and that it is all going to be fine, when it very well might not be. All my previous experience and the fact that I really do know my own body quite well tells me that what I have is malignant.

The very next day, I am out of school for the whole day at St Luke's Hospice for a strategy day with the board of trustees and the senior management team. I became a trustee three years before, specialising in fundraising – my marketing background being a useful skill as part of a multidisciplinary board.

It's funny how things happen, but I am obviously meant to hear something that is said that day. The consultant, Charles Daniels, another wonderful man who looked after my mum when she died at the Hospice in 2003, says a really important thing. He comments that when patients hear the word cancer, the first thing that springs to mind is death. Yet other patients, who are diagnosed with other much more debilitating diseases when told, do not have the same reaction. The reality, however, is that for most patients diagnosed with cancer the short term future is ropey, but the long term prognosis is often better and certainly gives a better quality of life in the long run than many other illnesses. It gets me to thinking that actually, if the diagnosis is cancer, then who am I to complain, when so many other people have such a worse quality of life and definitely have a much worse outlook. Breast cancer is, after all, very curable. One in three people will be diagnosed with cancer at some stage in their lives. Treatments have progressed so much that outcomes are far better than they were. Would I really rather have motor neurone disease, kidney failure or multiple sclerosis? You see, I told you I could find a silver lining in every cloud.

The next day, Friday, Zoe calls back and I tell her about the biopsy. (When Zoe tells Eamonn what I am calling about, and he had initially forgotten to tell her that I had called, he feels hugely guilty – he shouldn't. I told him it wasn't urgent.) I also tell my year group partner at school. I work with him so closely that it would be unfair not to. I also share it with a few other people who I am close to, especially the team I work directly with and two or three close friends. I don't want to worry them, but I know that I am not mentally firing on all cylinders at the moment and need them to understand why.

When you start to tell people about something as serious as this, you start to analyse your own behaviour. Well at least I do. I know not everyone reacts in the same way, as each individual will choose to handle how they manage such an issue on a very personal level. This is where the whole psychology of cancer begins. Because of the history that most people have with cancer and the uncertainty of the disease, you know that most people will have a negative reaction when told. I start to over process information. Do you tell people? If you do, why are you doing it? Will it worry them? If you don't tell them and they find out, how will they feel about the fact you didn't tell them? Are you telling them because you want sympathy? Definitely not! Well you don't think so? Argghhh. Stop thinking about it in so much detail – just do what feels right.

In case you haven't realised it by now, I am a bit of a control freak and also a workaholic. Both of these things in a good way of course! Coming into teaching later in life combined with my personality type means that I am passionate about my job and really care that it is done properly. The control freak in me is upset about the possibility of cancer because that is clearly totally out of my control. However, I am a realist and I also believe fervently that you should not worry about something that you cannot influence. So normality prevails as best it can.

CHAPTER 3

The Tests

Saturday morning comes and John has to take Marcus to see a prospective school, whilst Lizzie has to go to photography club followed by swimming. I go to the hospital for tests. First the mammogram. Now, for anyone who has ever had a mammogram you will know exactly what I am talking about, but for the uninitiated, let me explain the process.

You strip naked to the waist and sit in a gown and robe waiting for the radiographer. You are taken into the specific room where the instruments of torture await and you are briefed on what is going to happen. I already know, but I listen patiently. In turn, each breast is placed between two pieces of Perspex. The radiographer (who was fortunately female) manhandles (or in this case womanhandles) the breast into position, which means pulling the breast as far in-between the sheets of Perspex as possible. I actually think they are going to detach the breast from my chest at this point, which might mean I won't have to undergo a mastectomy if that is what the results show! When the breast is in place the two sheets of Perspex (which by the way are very cold) are slowly pushed as close together as possible by the radiographer. It is quite difficult to imagine how big a G cup breast can actually get and how thin it can become! Frisbee comes to mind at this point. Each breast is done horizontally and then at the diagonal vertically, so that they can get half of your armpit (where the lymph nodes are) at the same time. On the side where the lump is I nearly pass out with the pain and have to sit down with my head between my knees immediately afterward. Then I have a hot flush, just to top it all off (I am peri-menopausal, which means all the symptoms are in full swing, including hot flushes).

Since this episode, I have been sent an email about preparing for mammograms which is included here for amusement and to compare with the reality of the situation.

Mammograms

Many women are afraid of their first mammogram, but there is no need to worry. By taking a few minutes each day for a week preceding the exam and doing the following exercises, you will be totally prepared for the test and best of all, you can do these simple exercises right in and around your home.

EXERCISE ONE:
Open your refrigerator and insert one breast in door. Shut the door as hard as possible and lean on the door for good measure. Hold that position for five seconds. Repeat again in case the first time wasn't effective enough.

EXERCISE TWO:
Visit your garage at 3am when the temperature of the cement floor is just perfect. Take off all your clothes and lie comfortably on the floor, with one breast wedged under the rear tire of the car. Ask a friend to slowly back the car up until your breast is sufficiently flattened and chilled. Turn over and repeat with the other breast.

EXERCISE THREE:
Freeze two metal bookends overnight. Strip to the waist. Invite a

I FELT A RIGHT ONE...

stranger into the room. Press the bookends against one of your breasts.

Smash the bookends together as hard as you can. Set up an appointment with the stranger to meet next year and do it again.

YOU ARE TOTALLY PREPARED! (Anon)

I have to say that after receiving this, I laughed myself stupid – laughter is an important stress reliever, shifting as it often does on the hysterical border between laughter and crying.

So next, the biopsy. I am ushered into a warm, cosy room with one doctor and two nurses. The doctor explains that he would anaesthetise the breast with a small local injection. I did ask him why I could not have had this before the mammogram as it *really* would have helped. I show my chest to yet another group of total strangers. Perhaps I could have managed to be a topless model, because I have no embarrassment left anymore. It is just my body, a set of anatomical features and really just a large slab of meat ready to be examined.

Anyway, the doctor looks at the mammogram results but still needs to use the ultrasound to find where he is going to have to put the needle to collect the tissue sample. He has kindly warmed the gel, which gives him brownie points in my book when compared to the Surgeon! He then explains that he will be making a small hole through which he will angle a needle, from which he then fires another needle. Yes, you read it right, firing as in like a gun! This needle is then pulled out and takes a small slice (their term not mine) from the breast, which is called a core biopsy. I have to have four of these, with one aimed at the lymph nodes.

The doctor (who I have since discovered is the husband of a friend of a friend – Harrow is a very small place it seems) explains that the mammogram is not conclusive at all. In fact it is really hard to see the lump at all on the mammogram. He was suggesting that an MRI might also be needed. My memory is jogged about what

Karen, my friend in North Carolina, had said. I now decide to ask some of what I think are intelligent questions, including, "is there any relationship between size of breast and likelihood for malignancy?" The doctor answers that in fact, yes, there is and this is because the bigger the breast, the more breast tissue to potentially get diseased and also larger breasts also have more dense tissue, which is also more likely to produce cancer. I think *great* and wished I hadn't asked. Is ignorance bliss? No, not really, at least I am getting more information, which helps me feel like I am more in control, even though in reality I'm not.

The doctor is confirming my fears and is gently preparing me for the worst. He is kind, gentle, honest and very positive. I, by this stage, have decided on my management strategy, which is to be unerringly positive, with a tinge of realism. It is, all the time, looking more and more like cancer. So I talk non-stop to the poor doctor and nurses, thank them profusely, get dressed and go home.

Now the waiting starts. I know it is only for five days as I will get the results on Wednesday evening. The good thing is that John is in the country this week and will be coming with me to see Mr Burke, the surgeon, when he gives me either the good or bad news.

CHAPTER 4

The Results

I am only in school on Monday and Tuesday this week, as on Wednesday 1st October I am attending the first two days of a three day course on coaching and mentoring and I am really looking forward to it. The course is excellent and I get buddied up with a deputy head from another school and we have to practice coaching each other through a work related issue, using the non-directive method that we have been taught.

I have very few issues really, as my way of dealing with any problem in life is to sort it out as fast as you can. This normally involves someone in the senior management team being on the receiving end of a suggestion, question or proposed solution. So to try and find one for my buddy to facilitate solving is proving difficult. Also as I will find out the results of the tests that night, I am finding it a little difficult to focus on small work related issues when I may not even be at work for quite a while anyway! During the session I burst into tears on my buddy, but we laugh and still go through the process anyway.

That evening, before John comes home, whilst cooking dinner, I decide it is time to talk to Lizzie about the tests I have been having and what that might actually mean. I ask her if she knows what the tests are all about. Lizzie responds that she does. I probe a little deeper, but Lizzie says "I know what it is, but I don't want to say the word".

The Results

Lizzie is bright and has obviously already worked it all out. I can see she is worried and does not really want to talk about it, so I carry on cooking dinner. At least I know she is prepared and that she won't be shocked if the diagnosis is bad.

That night I have arranged for Sarah round the corner to have the children so that if the news is not good, we will have time to compose ourselves before having to talk to Lizzie and Marcus. I, thinking on the positive side, put a really good bottle of Taittinger champagne on ice in the fridge, ready to celebrate if it is good news.

John and I wait in the central waiting area. The fact that we are shown to the consultant's room rather than him coming to get us already indicates to me that the results are not going to be good. We sit down and the surgeon looks seriously at us both and says in a calm and gentle voice that he is sorry but it is not good news.

He goes on to explain that the biopsy has shown that there is a fairly extensive Lobular Carcinoma. This means that it is a multi focal cancer that is spread across an undetermined area of the right breast. Because of the type of cancer and the fact that the cells look quite like normal tissue (difficult little buggers) I need to have more tests to check the full extent of it. I need to have an enhanced MRI, which will also check if it is only in the right breast or has spread to the left as well. Thoughts begin to enter my mind about always wanting to have a breast reduction, it makes me giggle to myself and I know that I need to find all the silver linings that this rather large cloud has to offer.

I brightly ask if the priority is to save the breast. John looks at the surgeon and then at me as if I am totally mad (which I am, but that's another matter) and says, "No, it's to save your life Karen!"

I then comment jokingly that I had taken that as read! The good surgeon starts to talk about the possible treatment, and indicates that it is likely that I will need a full mastectomy of the right breast and depending on any spread, removal of the lymph nodes in the right armpit, probably chemotherapy and radiotherapy as well. John comments that I should not worry, because if I have a mastectomy

I FELT A RIGHT ONE...

and lose a breast, I "will still have more than most other women left in the other one alone."

I giggle (perhaps on the mildly hysterical side) and the surgeon looks a little strangely at us both. I think he is beginning to realise that we have a rather sick sense of humour. He does, however, to his credit remain serious and to the point.

This is a lot for both John and I to take in and I start babbling about telling everybody, thinking about my class and how much time I am going to have to take off school. Having only just gone full-time, I start to feel cross that I am going to have to miss time with my class. The kind surgeon says that he will get one of the nurses to take us somewhere and give us some more information to take home. He wants me to have an MRI on Saturday and come back and see him again next week. Then the extent of the cancer and the course of treatment can be discussed in more detail and timings can be decided.

John and I then meet a lovely nurse who is very sympathetic. She has obviously done this a hundred times and knows just what to say. John and I, although in shock, resort to our coping strategy of humour and start to make light of things. I am teary and still shocked, even though deep down I already knew. We decide to go home and open the champagne anyway. It seems a waste of electricity to have chilled it and then not drink it!

CHAPTER 5

Start Spreading the News

In the car on the way home, I call Sarah and Zoe to impart the bad news. As soon as it is time to tell other people, the reality of the diagnosis really starts to sink in and I get quite teary again.

John and I go home then sit and cry together at the kitchen table. We open the champagne and start to drink. We need to get ourselves together a bit before we go and collect the children from Sarah. After about half an hour, when we finally feel up to it we walk round the corner, have a quick drink with Sarah and Ed and bring the children home. We sit them down at the kitchen table.

I think Lizzie has already worked out what we want to talk about, but Marcus is totally clueless. We explain to both the children that I have been diagnosed with breast cancer but that they need to do more tests to discover the full extent and what the treatment will be. We explain about a mastectomy. Marcus starts to cry – as for him it is more of a shock – even though I am not sure he really understands what is going on, he just seems to know that he should be upset and so he is. Lizzie, however, starts to ask questions. I give them both a cuddle and answer all their questions (of which there are a lot) carefully. Marcus asks what would happen if I did not have the mastectomy, would they shrivel up and go black? We laugh at this and that breaks the atmosphere down as again humour comes to our rescue. I explain that an operation of some kind is essential otherwise the longer term outcome would be death.

Now John's sick sense of humour raises its head again. About three years ago I had a small skin cancer called a BCC (Basel Cell Carcinoma) removed from my face. This cancer is not a dangerous one and does not spread (metastasise), but just gets bigger and so still needs to be removed. At this point John gave me the nickname of 'cancer scabby face'. Yes, I know, what a lovely, affectionate turn of phrase my husband came up with. Anyway, John now turns to me and says, "What shall we call you now, 'cancer booby chest'?" The children and I totally collapse in mildly hysterical laughter.

With all this said and done, both children are shocked and more than a little upset. I ask if they would like their friends to know before tomorrow, so that when they go to school they have someone to talk to who knows why they might be upset. Also it is easier for me to tell people, than it is for them. They both say yes and I tell them I will phone their friends' parents so that they know.

The main difficulty for me is that Marcus goes to the school I teach at and so he has to keep it a secret for a while, until I have had a chance to tell the children in my class. I have already thought all this through and have decided that I want to be completely open about things. Living in the community close to the school in which I teach means that it will all come out in the open anyway and so I would like to manage the communication myself. Can you see the control freak strategy again?

I get on the phone and call three friends. Actually having to start telling people is hard. I have to be positive, but as I don't know all the answers yet, it is a difficult. But I have been thinking for a few weeks now what would happen if it turned out to be cancer and I have already decided how I am going to deal with it. Be matter of fact, unemotional if possible, which often depends on who you are telling, but most of all be positive.

If I am positive, then people will hopefully take their lead from me. If I am positive then they have to be positive too. If I am positive, it will be a signal to them to show them how I want to deal with this rather significant issue. If they react negatively then they may risk making me feel bad. I know that may sound really calculated, but I truly believe that you have to stay upbeat. Anyway, who wants to be around someone who is wallowing in self-pity? I don't. I have to live with me, remember.

When you tell someone that you have cancer, I think it is harder for them than it is for you. That may sound strange, but I believe it is true. The person who has cancer knows how they feel and is in full possession of all the information. They have already decided on how they want to manage it and have already, on a certain level, come to terms with their own personal situation and so are more in control. As soon as you tell someone else, although you have to deal with their emotions and how they handle your news, they are the ones who don't know what to say or how to react. They want to say and do the right thing and don't, under any circumstances, want to hurt your feelings. Then, you have to deal with their questions and you still don't have all the answers. The three friends are all shocked, saddened, but most of all fantastically supportive and will tell their children so that Lizzie and Marcus have someone who they can talk to in the morning. I also email Lizzie's form tutor to let her know.

The next morning, I go into school and go straight to Chris. Both he and the deputy head, Gill, are fantastic and give me a big hug each. We briefly discuss the way forward. They are both supportive of my decision that I would like to be totally open and tell my year group, so we decide to do it on the following Monday and send a letter out to parents. Chris will also tell all the staff at morning briefing. I am not going to be there as I am on the second day of the coaching/mentoring training course. I also walk up and see Marcus's teacher so that she knows. She is a colleague and I can see her getting upset on my behalf.

Why I want to be so open about having breast cancer may seem odd to some people, but for me there are multiple reasons. My parent's generation were definitely of the type that called it 'the big C'. It was a taboo and was not openly talked about, because in those days so many people died of cancer. As a teacher I am in a privileged position to influence how children think. By being open to all the children, it demystifies the disease for them and will hopefully make them realise that cancer is not a death sentence, but just a hiccup (if a fairly major one). If by my telling the children it stops one child having to worry about it so much in the future when they come across it again (which they will), then it will have been worth it.

Also, my work with St Luke's Hospice has taught me that cancer is not the worst disease that anyone can have. I am sure that different cancers affect the psychology of how you deal with it. Breast cancer has many connotations of how it will make you feel about your own body image, especially as a woman and especially with such a large chest! I want to try to help people realise this.

Remember as well that I live only 400m or so from the school that I teach at. I am part of the community, some of the children in my class live in my road, so they need to know. If they are going to see me walking round possibly bald from chemotherapy, then they need to understand why.

I also think that although I am a positive person, I actually benefit from the positive energy of others. If I tell people, then I am definitely going to get positive energy from some people and that can only be a good thing, right?

In the car on the way to the training course I talk to my colleague about what has happened. The more people you tell, the easier it gets. The second day of the course is better, as now the waiting and uncertainty are over; it is possible to start thinking of action plans and what is going to happen. A colleague on the course is the head of lower school at Lizzie's High School (the teaching community in Harrow is even closer than the rest of the community) and so I share the information, so it can be passed to all her teachers. The course leaders are very supportive and understanding and the day passes quickly.

On Friday it is back to school, where handling the response of lots of people becomes the issue. I am touched by people's concern and care and I am finding it easier and easier to talk about the cancer as more people approach me. A letter is drafted to parents ready for Monday.

At the weekend I start phoning several friends, including my best woman, Stevi, who now lives in Dubai. We as a family are due to go there for a week's holiday at half term (only three weeks away) and I need to warn her that we may have to change plans. I start to hope that we will still be able to go. I don't want to disappoint the children – I know they wouldn't think this, but I would hate for them to feel, even just a tiny bit, that they missed out on a great holiday because mum had cancer. This is not because I think that my children are selfish, they aren't, but they just don't understand the seriousness of issues in the same way that adults do. I also feel that a holiday before surgery as well as several more weeks in school will give me time to sort out my class and prepare to be 'off sick'. Others tell me I should not worry and that my health should come first, but I know what causes me stress. To have everything sorted and in order for the class before I go on sick leave will mean that I can relax a lot more whilst I am off.

The next week I have to go back for the final test: an enhanced MRI. This is what my friend Karen from North Carolina was talking about. A small cannula (needle that is inserted into a vein, generally on the back of your hand which is taped to you and has a little tap on it) is put into my right arm and a special fluid is then injected. This highlights the cancerous tissue in the breasts. I have to lie face down with my breasts dipped into two Perspex containers (at least this time they don't get flattened!) They give me some music to listen to and it takes about fifteen minutes.

I ask the radiographers if there is any chance I can find out whether the cancer has spread to the left breast. They both know why I am there and are very sympathetic. They go to see if the doctor who did the biopsy is there. He is and he takes both John and I into a small side room, where he puts the information onscreen and shows us there and then. There is nothing in the left

I FELT A RIGHT ONE...

breast (huge sigh of relief), but the right breast looks like it has a set of fairy lights all wrapped up around it.

The doctor confirms what I had already realised, which is that it will definitely be a mastectomy rather than a lumpectomy and the whole breast will have to come off.

At this moment I am grateful for private medical cover, as I am sure that if this had been on the NHS I would not have known the results until Wednesday, when I go to see the surgeon again. At least now I know and can start to get my head round what all this means.

As you know, I have made the decision to tell my class and in fact the whole year group, to which the head and deputy agreed. We do this on the Monday morning, after break, where we get all sixty children in the year group together in my class. There will be time at lunch to speak to any individual children who are affected if necessary. I have already phoned some parents of children in the class who I know personally, so that they are not shocked when they get the note that will go home with the children at the end of the day.

I have the support of the deputy and my year group partner as well as the two wonderful learning support assistants, Rowena and Kirti. I am honest and explain that I have breast cancer. I explain that I am going to have to have some time off for surgery, whilst I will have other treatment that might make me lose my hair and I will probably shave it off.

Some children burst into tears. There are lots of questions. Is cancer catching? Am I going to die? How long will I be away? Who is going to teach them? What is the operation going to be like? Gill and I answer the questions as best we can, with honest simplicity and most of the children seem to settle down. A handful need to spend some time with the deputy head outside the class as the rest settle down to work.

At lunchtime it spreads round the playground like wildfire and Marcus comes to me quite upset. Someone had come up to him and said, "Did you know Mrs Tighe has cancer?" How Marcus didn't punch them in the nose is quite surprising. He remained calm, but was still a little upset. I am really proud of him.

At the end of the day when the children take the letter out into the playground and immediately tell their parents, there are many individuals who want to speak to me. I am prepared for this and spend time talking to people, answering their questions and thanking them for their kindness. This is the least I can do. I am their children's teacher and there is going to be disruption for them. I have made the decision to be open and honest about what is wrong with me and I must therefore be prepared to put up with any reaction that comes my way. People are shocked, saddened, but amazingly supportive, which makes me feel I have done the right thing by being very open about it.

As I tell more and more people and have more and more detail to tell, I am starting to realise why I am doing this. By being open, having nothing hidden, by talking about it as if it is something that happens all the time (which of course it does, but just to lots of different people rather than just one), it makes cancer seem normal. That does seem ironic really, as there is nothing normal about cancer at all.

Cancer is mutated, abnormal cells that multiply and can spread through your body. However, feeling normal and in control is important to me and the more I talk about it, the more normal it feels. Others often don't know what to say to you or how to say it. If you say it for them, it may take away that awkwardness, makes them feel more at ease. I am sure that there are people who wish I wouldn't talk about it, but bless them they keep their thoughts to themselves, because they obviously realise that sharing is what I need to do.

A friend of mine, Ian (known as Hunty), had testicular cancer over twenty years ago. He writes a wonderful card to me and makes some really interesting points. He comments that although you would never wish to have cancer, you end up being on the receiving end of this huge wave of love, support and good wishes. This is truly an amazing gift to be given and one that you would never know was out there unless you became seriously ill. Hunty also writes about how it is for the partner of a cancer sufferer – "The person closest to you will also be feeling the most helpless – almost a bystander, with his nose pressed up against the window, desperately looking for ways to make it better and most often only feeling that 'if only I could do more.'"

Reading this is helpful, if a little emotional, for both John and I. I keep every card, letter, note and email that people send me, as the blanket of warmth, kindness and generosity of heart makes you feel really supported and special. Not special in a negative, 'people are feeling sorry for me' way, but in a loved, 'people care about what happens to me' way.

CHAPTER 6

So What's the Treatment?

When you get diagnosed with cancer, you are given lots of information leaflets from Cancerbackup. They are well worth reading and have lots of really good advice. One of the pieces of advice that I will take on board is to write down any questions that I want to ask. I get a notebook and start to write. You have so many unanswered questions in your head and you know that if you don't write them down then you'll forget them. I don't write down the answers, just the questions.

So a couple of days later on Wednesday 8th October, John and I return to see the lovely surgeon and talk through the results of the MRI and what that means for decisions about my treatment. As suspected it means a full mastectomy of the right breast, but to determine if the cancer has spread to the lymphatic system I need to have something called a sentinel node biopsy. This is where they inject some radioactive material into the breast and track where the material circulates to, which then shows the key lymph node. This will be removed at the beginning of the mastectomy operation and taken away for testing whilst I am in surgery, the results come back before the end of the operation. If the tests show that there are cancerous cells, it will determine how many other lymph nodes are removed in addition to the breast tissue.

We discuss planned timings of the surgery which is pretty

critical, as I am really keen not to miss our holiday in Dubai. The surgeon is happy that we have the holiday and arranges the surgery for 12th November – five days after my forty-seventh birthday and the week after we return from Dubai. He says the cancer is a slow progressing one, but prescribes a drug called Tamoxifen to start taking straight away. This drug is something I am likely to have to take for five years after all the other treatment is finished. I must also, when I fly, wear compression stockings (to protect against the risk of a deep vein thrombosis – DVT) mmm sexy! And I must take one aspirin to thin my blood, one day before flying.

My cancer is probably hormone receptive to both oestrogen and progesterone. The Tamoxifen blocks the hormone receptors in the cancer cells. Because the hormones are likely to promote tumour growth, taking the drug should reduce any further spread.

As well as the surgery, the surgeon talks about the likely follow-up treatment – almost certainly a course of chemotherapy and perhaps radiotherapy as well. He keeps calling me a 'young woman with breast cancer', which makes me feel quite chuffed! No one has called me that in a long time and being a primary school teacher, the children definitely think of you as old! It still seems like so much to take in and it feels like the treatment is going to take such a long time. The surgeon comments that you really have to write off about a year of your life. How *bloody inconvenient,* I think.

Believe it or not I am already interested in reconstructive surgery, as I cannot imagine walking around lopsided for the rest of my life. I mention that I am worried about walking round in circles. The surgeon replies with a smile, saying that it wouldn't happen, but that I might end up leaning a bit! I am also very much in the frame of mind that there will be a 'rest of my life'. This is, I feel, just a blip; a hurdle to overcome and then I can get on with the rest of my life as normal.

The surgeon talks through some basic types of reconstructive surgery and says he approves of looking up this kind of information on the internet, but not stuff about the cancer itself. He counsels that spending time on the internet to find out about the disease is counterproductive, as all it does is confuse and worry. Everyone is different and individual so you never know what information you are going to come across. I have already decided not to look at the internet anyway, but am happy to read all the literature that the doctors and nurses have given me from Cancerbackup and MacMillan.

I am now allowed to go away until just before the operation to enjoy life, have a holiday and get myself straight at school before taking time off. The surgeon says that I should rest for at least six weeks after the surgery but that I can start chemo after about three weeks, which would take another four months, and then possibly onto radiotherapy… Here comes the year out of my life.

I am really glad of the time before the operation. I really feel it is giving me space to get my head straight and come to terms with what is happening to me. Because of my completely open coping strategy, people are generally treating me like me, not like a person with cancer. This desire for normality is really pushing me to be as upbeat as possible.

Over the next couple of weeks things start to settle down, but an amazing thing happens. People start to give you things; books mostly, self help and alternative medicine books. But the most precious gift of all is people's kindness and support. Letters and cards continue to arrive with such incredibly kind words of support that I am overwhelmed by how much people care.

I have emailed most of my friends abroad as I don't want them to have a shock when they get the annual newsletter and Christmas card, which will bear the news. Friends start phoning from Canada, New Zealand and the US. I get used to repeating the same information and am starting to get a little tired of talking about cancer all the time, but I know that by doing it this way, it will get it all over and done with more quickly.

After a couple of weeks it becomes apparent that many children in the school, who I have taught in the past, are concerned about me. The learning mentors, who support children with behavioural and social issues in our school, come and tell me that they are getting a lot of children coming and talking to them about me. I consult with Gill and Chris and suggest that when I deliver my middle school assembly this week, I should also talk to them about myself.

I do, and the children listen very attentively. I arrange for Marcus to spend some time with his teacher, so that he does not have to sit there and listen to me give this assembly. It would be hard for him, as all the other children would look for his reaction. I tell them that I am going to shave my head before my hair starts to fall out and ask the children if they will sponsor me. Every child puts their hand up and I very nearly burst into tears.

CHAPTER 7

The Calm Before the Storm

At the end of October we, as a family, fly to Dubai to stay with Stevi, her husband Brian and their daughter Katie. Everyone has a great time and I am so pleased to spend some time with one of my closest friends who I don't get to see too much anymore. Stevi has organised a camping trip in the desert, which, considering that two of the things I hate most in the world are camping and sand, is not something I am looking forward to!

We do camp and as a trick Brian and John conspire to put sand in my sleeping bag. Of course they have to put it in John's sleeping bag as well, because otherwise I will know it is John's idea. What they didn't bank on is that I get a case of the galloping trots and have to keep going off into the dunes with a spade and roll of toilet paper all evening to sort myself out. All in the camp knew the trick had been set, but when I go to bed I don't get in the sleeping bag as it is too hot. Only in the middle of the night, after a visit to another sand dune, do I actually get into the sleeping bag and discover the sand. I wake John and ask him if he has sand in his bag too and he confirms that he does. We get up, empty the sand outside and go back to sleep.

In the morning I accost Brian, who tells me it had been John's idea. I begin to plot revenge. In fact before breaking camp, I fill a Ziploc bag with sand to bring back to the UK to wreak revenge over

I FELT A RIGHT ONE...

a period of time. Little does John know what is going to hit him!

Before we leave Dubai Brian gives me a wonderful present: a full range of Harley Davidson headgear, containing all sorts of different headscarves that are really cool. How thoughtful and generous. I tell him I will wear them with pride. Stevi gives me an early birthday present of pyjamas, slippers and a dressing gown, so that I will be able to look fabulously glamorous whilst in hospital.

Returning from Dubai, I have lots to get ready in this last week at school. I work with the supply teacher who is going to take the class over until Christmas; I hand over my other work, as well as going for all the final tests, buying pyjamas and soft bras. I have measurements taken of my right arm so that they can be checked in future for any swelling in the arm on the side of the mastectomy.

One of the potential side effects of having lymph nodes removed is that the body's ability to manage the removal of fluid which it uses to protect itself from an injury or infection is significantly reduced. This can, in the future, create something called lymphoedema, or the swelling of the arm on the side of the mastectomy.

I meet with the breast care nurse, Elaine, who is wonderful, and for the first time since originally being told I have cancer, I cry. I am able to talk to someone about what worries me most. How will I feel without a breast? What will it look like? Will it be completely flat? The nurse answers all my questions and I am actually able to articulate for the first time how worried I am about what I will feel about my own body after the operation. Will I still feel like a woman? Will I still feel attractive? Having such a large chest has often caused me problems, particularly for sport and buying clothes. What is it going to be like afterwards? Will John still love me in the same way when I only have half of what I know he likes most about me physically? I know that I will no longer be able to wear underwired bras and that I obviously will no longer have a cleavage. I talk it through with Elaine and I feel more prepared for what is to come.

The Calm Before the Storm

Finally I am ready. My last day in school is also my forty-seventh birthday and at the weekend we have a group of some of our oldest and closest friends round for dinner. This evening had been arranged months before and I am pleased to be enjoying time with good friends and just being as normal as possible. We always laugh a lot and this evening is no exception.

The day before the operation I go to hospital to have the radioactive injection and the scan to find the sentinel node, so that tomorrow when the surgeon is operating he will be able to find the prime node to remove to be checked to see if the cancer had spread. This is another learning curve in medical procedures for me. Having one's nipple injected with radioactivity is quite painful and a sensation that I would be pleased to not have to repeat. The good thing is that after the operation I am only going to have one nipple left, so that reduces the likelihood by 50%!

After the injection I have to lie still whilst the person (I am now losing track of who all the different people are that I am dealing with and am I not sure if he is a doctor, radiographer, radiologist, nurse, technician or what – but I have since discovered that he is a physicist!) using a special scanner tracks and plots where the radioactivity has travelled to. When the scanning is complete, the radiographer produces a picture that clearly shows where the main lymph node providing the drainage system for my right breast is. The surgeon now has his road map for finding the sentinel node.

CHAPTER 8

The Operation

Tuesday 12th November has come around so quickly. The six weeks since diagnosis have just flown by. I have to be at the hospital at 7.30am and John is going to spend the day with me. In fact John's boss Ray has been fantastic and luckily John is in the country for this week and the next one.

Now, do you remember the sand I collected and surreptitiously brought back from Dubai? Zoe, my sister-in-law, had a cunning plan, which was that on the morning of going into hospital, I should get my revenge on John with the sand. So, as John is downstairs putting my bag in the car, I flip back the duvet and using the bag of sand sprinkle the words 'I love u' onto the bed. The thought that when John gets home, tired and fed up from being with me all day in hospital, he will go to bed, only to find that he has to change the sheets first, keeps my spirits up no end. Everyone knows except John. It really cheers me up and will teach him a lesson as well!

I feel lucky thanks to John having private medical insurance that I am going to a private hospital. Not that it makes much difference to the treatment you receive, but does, however, mean that I have been able to have all my appointments at my convenience. Evenings and weekends mostly, so I miss less time at school and cause less disruption for the children. It also means that I know I will sleep better, as I will have a room to myself.

The Operation

We arrive as required at 7.30am, then get checked in as I am due to go to surgery at 8.30am. I get undressed and then redress into the gown and paper knickers (yes, you heard it, paper knickers). The lady anaesthetist comes to visit, then the surgeon comes to visit and I complete all the required paperwork and consent forms.

I am taken down to surgery, chatting all the way. Poor staff, just what they need early in the morning, a garrulous patient who cannot keep quiet. All I can think about is how many lymph nodes I will wake up with. What will that sentinel node show? Will the cancer have spread?

At this point I also need to tell you something that Zoe said. Zoe used to be a chemotherapy nurse and when I first started talking to her about having cancer she described what it does to you, in the psychological sense, as a 'Head F**k'. She is so right, because the disease is so unpredictable, everyone is different and you never know when, or if, it is going to come back, so it completely messes with your head. I am just at the beginning of this journey and the first hurdle I have to overcome will be the results of surgery and what it shows.

I am wheeled into the operating theatre, where the anaesthetist works her magic and I wake up in recovery asking for my glasses. It really is the strangest sensation, having a general anaesthetic, as hours could have gone by and you just don't know it. I am taken back up to my room, where John has been waiting patiently for a couple of hours. I feel strange. I have two cannulas in my left hand; one for intravenous fluids and one for morphine (PCA – patient controlled analgesia – pain relief drugs). From the right hand side of my body are two tubes draining fluid from the wound. Both my legs have compression stockings on and are also attached to pumps which keep contracting and relaxing, so as to keep the blood moving round my legs and minimise the risk of a DVT. To top it off I also have an oxygen mask on, as the nurses tell me that morphine lowers your respiration and so they have to do this to help keep my blood oxygen level up. I feel like something out of a horror film and I

I FELT A RIGHT ONE...

wonder how on earth I am going to go to the loo!

The most pressing thing on my mind is knowing how many lymph nodes have been taken. I will have to wait till the surgeon comes, but I am desperate to find out. I peek down under the gown and my chest looks incredibly flat; what had I expected, they have taken my rather large breast off. Nevertheless, I am surprised at just how much tissue has been taken; my chest almost looks concave on the right side. I had never realised how far breast tissue actually extends into your body. The fact that I am so large on the other side seems to make it worse. The good thing is that I don't mind looking at it, because I had thought that I would be upset and I had thought I would feel less of a woman. I had thought that it would frighten me, but at the moment I don't seem to mind. Maybe it's the drugs.

I am starving so they bring me a cup of tea and a biscuit. I am not in too much pain, but I keep myself dosed up with morphine. These machines are clever and only let you have a certain amount every ten minutes or so. The nurses track how many times you request some drugs and how many times the machine has actually administered it. This way the nurses know how much pain you are likely to be in. John sits quietly, working at his PC and reading the newspaper whilst I doze.

Then the physioterrorist comes to visit. Yes, can you believe it, but she wants to check that I can sit up, cough and generally move around. The minute I sit up I feel sick and start to throw up. Luckily there is only a small amount of tea and biscuit to get rid of, but I keep retching all the same. The nurse says it could be the morphine. I remember back to how my mum had been really sick with morphine and also when I had the disc taken out of my neck, how sick I had been then. I had always assumed it had been the anaesthetic. I put two and two together and decide that it is definitely the morphine making me sick, so I stop pressing the button. The nurses quickly get an anti-sickness drug and give me an injection in bottom. The word pin-cushion comes to my mind at this point, but I don't care as long as I stop being sick. Very quickly I do. Yippee.

The Operation

As the morphine wears off I can stop wearing the oxygen mask and I also realise that I am really not in too much pain after all.

That afternoon the surgeon comes to see John and I. He tells us that they found cancer in the sentinel node and so he has removed all the major lymph nodes on the right side (about twenty to twenty three). This, he explains, is significant. He talks about how for the rest of my life I will have little feeling under the armpit of that arm (as the nodes are inextricably wrapped up with the second brachial intercostal nerve, which thus gets severed) and also that I should never have any injections or blood pressure taken on that arm due to the risk of lymphodoema, as I mentioned before. The fluid builds up in the arm as there is no effective drainage system anymore because the lymph nodes have been removed. He tells me that the physio will give me details of what not to do and suggests that when cleaning or gardening gloves should always been worn, also that I need to be careful when having manicures as well. I didn't want to get a scratch that could get infected and make my whole arm swell up. Deep joy!

I feel a little cross; as if having a breast removed is not enough, now I have to deal with all this crap about lymphodoema. In fact, the worst of the pain is not actually in the chest, but down the arm from where the nerves have been cut. I think this to myself, as I am sure that if I express how I feel to anyone then they will think I am mad. So what if you get a swollen arm and some pain? You don't have cancer anymore. The difficulty is that the cancer itself has little actual impact on your life (apart from the mastectomy of course!) but all the consequences of the treatment give you a large range of issues to deal with. I am also now worried about whether the cancer had spread. It is not good news that he has found cancer in the sentinel node. How many other nodes are affected? Has it spread still further? Head f**k time again!

With all the fluids being delivered intravenously, I need the loo. The nurses kindly bring me a bed pan, but it is too awkward on the bed with all the tubes and stuff. They then bring in a commode,

I FELT A RIGHT ONE...

detach the leg pumps, help me lift the drainage bottles over and sit down. It really is the strangest sensation to be desperate for the loo, but not be able to go. I sit and sit but my muscles cannot relax enough to let go. Boy, I wish it was like this normally; my pelvic floor has never really recovered from having two children and I usually have to make mad dashes to the loo. Today it is the complete opposite. Bless them, the nurses even try running the taps in the bathroom.

I order dinner and John makes sure that I have no visitors that day so that I get lots of rest. The more rest I get, the quicker I will recover. He is like a guard dog, being so protective and I love him for it. He finally leaves to go home at about 7.30. Now I can cheer myself up with the thought of him going home to see the children and then having to change the sheets before going to bed! How will he react? I do hope he sees the funny side of my practical joke. He calls at about 10.30 and has still not been upstairs to our bedroom. I don't say anything as I don't want to spoil the shock and annoyance. One has to take small pleasures in times of desperation, especially in the name of revenge.

The next day my hand is getting sore and swollen from the cannulas and as I don't need the pain relief or fluids, they take them out. They also take off the leg pumps and I am able to get up. One of the nurses, Cleo, helps give me a shower. Wow, I feel a million dollars. Something as simple as a shower can have such a significant impact on your wellbeing. I feel human again.

John comes in early and I can hear the nurse ask him how he slept. He now knows that everyone else knew about my trick; that makes it even better. He did see the funny side of it and could not believe that I had been so devious. Even the surgeon when he comes to see me later asks him how he had slept. I laugh out loud this time.

John stays with me all day then goes home to get Lizzie and Marcus from school and brings them up to see me. We have waited until I am not plugged into so many things as we don't want to frighten them too much. It is so lovely to see them and I think they are relieved to see me so well and cheerful.

Children will take their lead from you. They don't know how to react to circumstances unless you give them an indication. I also think that my children would want to behave in the right way in case they upset me, but I want them to see that I am really OK, both physically and emotionally. Whilst they are visiting, Lizzie shows me the photo she had taken of the 'I love u' that I had written on the bed in sand. What a fantastic thought. It gives me even more pleasure to retell the story and show the evidence. I am not sure that people really believed I had done it, but when they saw the photo they realise that I actually did. As the saying goes, laughter is the best medicine, and this particular prescription was proving to be very beneficial.

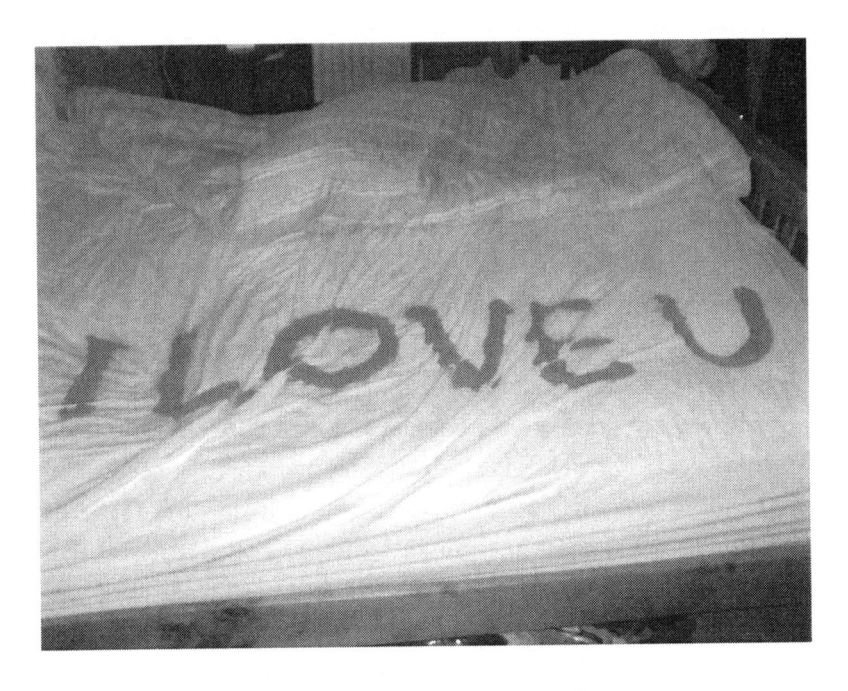

Photo courtesy of Lizzie Tighe

I FELT A RIGHT ONE...

Over the weekend I have lots of fantastic visitors. My lovely nephew (age twenty-seven), who would normally be out partying on a Friday night, spends a couple of hours keeping me company, which is fun. School colleagues, family and friends all come to see me. I like to get up and walk out with them so I can get the exercise and so they can see how well I am. I feel great and I want everyone to know it. I am sure that I am trying to show people that I can manage; that I am OK and that in some way I am also trying to prove it to myself! One colleague thought I wanted him to leave when I offered to walk him to the door. I am obviously not making myself clear. I blame the anaesthetic!

On Sunday the drains are taken out and the surgeon says I can go home tomorrow. Barbara the physio comes to see me with what she fondly calls a 'comfy'. A comfy is basically a breast shaped cushion. John is with me when she visits and casually asks what sizes they come in. I suggest that one of the larger sizes is going to be required! She gives me a size ten, which is not actually the largest, but almost. I try it for size. I slip it inside my bra and with clothes on you would hardly notice the difference. In the pack there is some extra padding which you can add into the back of the comfy as it gets flattened down over time. I will have to wear this for about six weeks, or until my wound has settled down enough to have something more substantial pressing against it. I have bought some soft bras in preparation for this, which feels really strange as I have been wearing underwired bras for the last twenty-five years.

Barbara also gives me my booklet about all the exercises I need to do to keep the right side of my body working properly. The mastectomy and loss of skin over the chest makes the range of movement in my right arm much reduced. The scar tissue also tightens over time and so you need to exercise to make sure you don't end up with one arm that can do a lot less than the other. You know at this point, I really think I am lucky. Imagine how I would feel if I had ended up losing both breasts with a double mastectomy.

That night John goes home and sends out an email update. He

The Operation

has been sending them out when there has been some news. It saves lots of phone calls and means that all the wonderful people who care about me are in the loop. By the way, you need to know that my nickname is Motey. Everyone calls me that as my maiden name was Mote, even my nephews and nieces call me Aunty Motey!

(Note sent on Sunday 16.11.08 entitled – Motey home tomorrow – Hooray)

Dear all

Motey had her drains removed this afternoon and has progressed well enough that she will come home tomorrow (Monday) to REST!!!

We all know that Karen is not very good at resting, so I will need support from you in ensuring she does not launch herself into redecorating bedrooms and landscaping the garden while she recuperates. Tidying up and making tea all the time might be lesser evils but I also want her to avoid these, at least for the next week. We will hopefully get a better feel for the timing of the next steps later in the week, but her wound does have to be completely healed before chemo.

Please do visit/send messages/phone when you are able, but be sympathetic to ensuring Karen gets rest and if she is sleeping please do not feel offended if she does not answer a door or return a phone call straight away. If visiting in person please feel free to make YOURSELVES tea/coffee etc.

Thank you all for your good wishes,
Johnny

As you can see, John is being very protective of me, which some of my friends say made them cry when they read it. Reading it back now makes me a little emotional too.

By Monday mid morning I am ready to rock and roll. I have asked John to bring in some thank you cards from home. He has

I FELT A RIGHT ONE...

also bought some chocolates and hand cream. You can never give nurses too much hand cream as a present; think how many times a day they wash their hands and imagine how dry they get. I sit and write a thank you note to all the staff on the ward and an individual note to Cleo.

I think that you often bond with people in times of difficulty and I find that I have bonded with Cleo. A mature, wise, kind and gentle natured woman, whose chosen vocation means that people like me get treated with such great care. The surgeon has warned me that although I am an incredibly positive person, I will have my down times and he is right. During my stay in hospital there is one night, where for some reason, I feel really alone and lost (one of the negatives of private care is that it can get very lonely in a single person room). The next morning I have a long chat to Cleo about it. She totally understands. Her ability to listen and be empathetic without having had the same personal experience comes out of her years of experience. She has worked with Mr Burke for many years and so had cared for a large number of breast cancer patients. Cleo knows what to say and when to say it.

John has to make a few trips to the car, as my room now resembles a florist. In just a few days I have more bunches of flowers and arrangements than I can ever remember receiving before in one go. People are so thoughtful and, you know, flowers really do cheer you up. They brighten up any room and are a physical and visual reminder of the care and thoughts that people are having for you.

With a happy goodbye, we are off home. Only four nights in hospital – not bad going I think. I am so happy to be going home, as this marks the next stage of my recovery and treatment. I have an appointment during the week to see the surgeon again to get the results of the tests on my lymph nodes, so I know there is still a long way to go, but this is a good start.

CHAPTER 9

Recuperation

We go home, but that afternoon is going to be the first parent meeting with Lizzie's tutor at high school. I do not want to miss it and am keen to go. I know I have just come out of hospital, but apart from walking slowly I don't see a problem with going. We drive to school and go to the meeting. Normality is resuming!

One of the first things I do when I get home is write a thank you letter to Michael Burke. What do you say to someone who has saved your life? I know that may sound a little melodramatic, but it is the truth; by removing the cancer, he has undoubtedly saved my life. It is not just the fact that he has had to support me through probably the hardest issue I am likely to face in my life, but also that he is genuinely an incredibly good man – so wise and knowledgeable. He has seen hundreds of women like me, in fact he treated both my mum and a sister-in-law. I take my time and craft the letter, so that I can truly express to him how grateful I am. Thousands of doctors work extraordinarily hard, I am sure often to the detriment of their families. However, the benefits that the patients gain are immeasurable.

Over the next couple of weeks, whilst I am unable to drive I spend a lot of time having coffee and chatting to friends. Stevi is over from Dubai (a visit she has purposefully timed for now) and comes to see me a couple of times. Some friends are regular visitors, which makes the days pass quickly. The week after I come out of hospital John is away again and different friends come round and cook or drop some dinner in. Rowena and Kirti, the two learning support assistants that I work with come to see me and I realise how much I miss their company at school.

John is away again the following week and before he goes, I tamper with his shampoo and add some more of the Dubai sand, in the hope that it might give him an exfoliating head rub. Can you believe it, he doesn't even notice. The sand sinks to the bottom of the shampoo bottle and has absolutely no effect. I am totally gutted. However, John was in Egypt and he brings back his own bottle of sand so that a truce can be called.

Being the obsessively organised person that I am, I find it difficult to ask for help or even to just accept it. But, you know, I discover a wonderful thing: people really do want to help. They will do anything they can for you. This has two major benefits. You do need help after such a major operation and friends are desperate to feel better about your situation. Doing something practical is something concrete which they can do to help. In fact there is a third benefit for us, which is that because John is away so much of the time, he is really worried that I will overdo things. All these friends helping really makes sure that I don't. So you see, another silver lining to the cloud, as I learn how to graciously accept help from others. I learn that it is important to both parties, but most amazingly I learn how kind so many different people are.

Two days after coming out of hospital, John and I go back to visit the surgeon. This is crunch time. We get to find out the likelihood of the cancer having spread. We go back on the Wednesday evening and wait patiently to be shown into his room. As we are ushered in, Michael Burke stands up and shakes both our hands, and then sits down.

"Good news," he says with a slight smile. The pathology report on all the lymph nodes removed (twenty-three in total) shows no sign of any cancerous cells except the sentinel node itself, the original one that he took out at the very beginning of the surgery. The cancer in this node was 5mm in width, so not tiny. However, the fact that it was only in this one node meant that the cancer should not have spread to anywhere else in my body. No secondary metastatic cancer.

The pathology results also include the results of the hormone receptor tests. The cancer is tested for its reaction to the hormones oestrogen, progesterone and herceptin. The results are scored out of eight. My cancer was 7/8 receptive for oestrogen, 4/8 for progesterone and not receptive at all to herceptin. These results are important for the planning of longer term treatment.

The cancer only being in the sentinel node is highly significant, so to say I am relieved at this point, is probably the understatement of the year. I want to jump for joy, but I reign myself in. John smiles as the enormity of the positive news sinks in.

So now we have the discussion as to what the next course of treatment is to be. Michael (yes, I did ask if I could call him that) tells us that it is now time to refer me to the oncologist that he works with – David Fermont, who has also treated my mum and my sister-in-law.

Michael says he will see me again in three months. We talk about the fact that I will need to start chemotherapy as soon as I can, which is normally about three weeks after the original operation. I need to wait until the wound is fully healed, as chemotherapy, reduces the body's ability to heal. I need to have the chemo, because even though he is confident that the cancer has not spread, it is a belt and braces approach. This will ensure that any erroneous cancer cells wandering around my body will get nuked! The most reassuring thing that Michael says during the whole visit is that I am a young woman "who has *had* breast cancer," meaning that I no longer have it. He has surgically removed it all and any further treatment that I now have is 'just in case'.

During this visit we end up talking about all sorts of aspects such as how I feel, the treatment etc, but Michael also touches on some really interesting points. He can see that I am keen to go full pelt into everything so that I can sort my life out and he counsels wisely about a few things. One is that I have to let my body take its time to get better, that I need to be kind to myself and listen to my body. The second is about how other people see me.

He talks about the longer term. How will I feel when I am no longer the centre of attention? He comments that some people find that although they did not really want the limelight, they quite enjoy it whilst they have it. Adjusting to not being the focus of peoples' thoughts can be a bit of an anti-climax after the life-threatening illness you have had. You will always think back to it and have to manage the longer term side effects of the treatments, however, after a while most other people will forget (which to me seems a good thing) and life will go back to normal. How will I cope when this happens? Again, an interesting view of the psychological effects of cancer that I had not considered. I think I can honestly say that I don't think this will be a problem. My outgoing personality means that I often crave attention and behave in a way that demands it. Being a teacher I get the opportunity every day at work – I think my class pays attention most of the time!

More importantly, he comments that even after you are well and definitely clear of cancer, other people can still see you as a cancer sufferer. They still worry about you. He talks about how at some time in the future, if you feel unwell or have a recurring ache or pain, you have to put up with some of the people closest to you looking at you in a way that means they are worried about whether it is cancer again. He describes it as 'when do I become Karen again and not Karen who had cancer'. An interesting thought. That night when I get home I send out an update email myself.

I find that whilst I am stuck not driving so soon after surgery, the lifeline of emails is fantastic, especially with some of my good friends who live abroad. Word gets around to friends with whom contact had become rare and sporadic and they start emailing me as well. It really keeps me in a positive frame of mind to be in contact with so many friends. If you cannot see them in person then the virtual contact, although a poor substitute, is better than nothing.

The next day I find myself chatting to Lizzie in the kitchen whilst she helps me make dinner – slight over-exaggeration – rather reheating a ready meal. I am telling her about the importance of the pathology results and I ask her, "Have you been worried about me?"

"What would you do if I said no?" was her instant response.

At this point I am thinking of the old adage, which is never ask a question that you don't want to hear the answer to. I then reply, "Well I would thank you for your honesty and say that your father and I did absolutely the right thing in being totally honest with you and Marcus." The way we had decided to deal with my having cancer, matter of fact, open, honest – no conversations behind closed doors – means that I have never shown my children that I am frightened, so therefore they aren't either.

I am glad that Lizzie can be so honest with me about how she feels as well. She makes me laugh when she says, "Do you know, Mum, if one more random adult who I would never normally speak to says to me 'If you need to talk to someone, I am always here for you', I am going to scream. Don't they realise that if I am worried I will talk to you, dad or someone vaguely close to me?"

Some close friends are being particularly supportive and we go out for 'girls' beers'. Our husbands regularly do this, but for some reason we don't seem to get to out as often. These girls know me so well, one since I was twenty. They can say anything to me and often do! A sign of true friendship. I get to talking about when my hair is going to fall out and suggest that I could shave it off in an assembly at school. They are not so sure, especially because of how it might make Marcus feel. What would happen if I got upset in front of the children? They are right of course, but sometimes I don't like hearing "no".

Although I am signed off from work I am starting to get bored and so attend a couple of training/professional development events to keep my brain ticking over. On 28th November John and I go to

I FELT A RIGHT ONE...

visit David Fermont, the oncologist.

He greets us warmly and says that now the surgery is over and the cancer has been removed, he is my 'insurance policy'. His words, not mine. I like the sound of this. He makes it all sound so easy.

He tells us that I will have to have six chemotherapy treatments on a drug regimen called FEC (to me this sounds like an Irish swear word). FEC is an acronym for the three different drugs that make up the cocktail I will be receiving; F for Fluoroucil, also known as 5FU, E for Epirubicin and C for Cyclophosphadmide. I will have to have this every three weeks. Chemotherapy works at a systemic level on your whole body. It is very clever and only attacks the cells that are dividing in your body. The problem is that it attacks any cell in your body that is dividing; in your mouth, muscles, hair, stomach, everywhere. This is why your immune system will be negatively affected, as all the good cells in your body that are multiplying to protect you get destroyed too.

I will also have to have a course of radiotherapy. David comments that there have been studies looking at the effectiveness of short-course radiotherapy (fifteen doses) for women with under five lymph nodes affected with cancer and he says it is a 'no-brainer' and I should just have it done. Finally, I will need to take Tamoxifen for five years, or another drug which inhibits the uptake of hormones to reduce the likelihood of any recurrence of the cancer.

We arrange a time to go and meet Mary the chemo sister to get weighed, measured and briefed about all the side effects that the drugs can give. David tells us that he will see me any time I feel I need to during chemo, but definitely after the third round. We chat a little while longer and when I tell him that I intend to shave my hair off to raise money for St Luke's Hospice, it transpires that we also have a lot in common as he used to be on the board of trustees a few years before.

A couple of days later I return to the hospital to meet Mary and also Rommel, who is in charge of my induction and takes me off to be weighed and measured. This needs to be done so that they can get the correct dose of the wonderfully poisonous drugs. He then sits down to brief me on all the side effects that chemo can cause. The list is long:

- Lowered resistance to infection
- Bruising or bleeding
- Anaemia (low number of red blood cells)
- Feeling and being sick
- Tiredness
- Hair loss
- Sore mouth and ulcers
- Taste changes
- Skin changes
- Irritation of the bladder
- Diarrhoea
- Constipation
- Gritty eyes and blurred vision
- Changes in nails
- Changes in the way your heart works
- DVT
- Affects on fertility
- Loss of periods (is that such a bad thing at my age?)
- Leakage of the drugs into the skin around your vein

I know there is a view that if you know all this, it might make you think some of these things are happening when actually they aren't. If you look for the side effects, will it make them appear? However, at least if you know what might happen then you won't be surprised and as the saying goes, forewarned is forearmed.

The most important issue we discuss is whether I want to reduce the likelihood of hair loss. One can have something called a cold cap, which cools the scalp and reduces the blood supply to the hair follicles and so reducing the damage to this part of your body. The problems with this are that apparently it is quite uncomfortable to wear and can make the chemo take longer to give. There is also a really tiny chance that if a cancer cell has spread to your scalp, then it won't be destroyed. To me, if I am going to all this trouble, I may as well go the whole hog. I have decided to shave my hair off to raise money for St Luke's anyway, and if I have the scalp cooling then there would be no point in doing that.

For some people I am sure that the thought of losing their hair is frightening and they may feel that it makes their treatment too public, when they want to keep what they are going through more private. I completely respect and understand this, but seeing as I am at the other end of the spectrum I think going bald is not going to be a problem.

Now I am fully prepared for the chemo, with the first session being scheduled for Thursday 4th December. During this time period I am voraciously reading all the books I have been given – partly because I have little else to do and also because if people have been kind enough to give them to me, then they must think they are worth reading. So, why not? I read one called *The Secret* by Ronda Byrne first. This is a book all based on the laws of attraction. In summary it suggests that if you think positively about something, then what you are thinking about will happen and conversely if you are thinking about something negatively, it will also happen. Just the fact that your mind is focussing on the topic means whatever you are mentally directed at will increase the incidence or likelihood of it happening.

When applying the theory to me, I am pretty sure that I have never thought *I want breast cancer*. I don't even really think I had thought too much of *I don't want breast cancer*. Breast cancer was not something I had ever thought about in relation to me, only in relation to others. Could I have got cancer because I like being the centre of attention? However, any thoughts of being the focus of attention I have considered in the past were always about being socially adept, more aimed at telling a good joke and making people laugh than getting cancer. Cancer does not normally make people

Recuperation

laugh. This thought also makes me consider what Michael Burke had said about coping later on, when you are no longer the focus of people's thoughts. I can honestly say that I am really looking forward to being 'normal' again, the being 'just Karen'.

I next read a book called *The Journey*, by Brandon Bays. This book was given to me by the parent of a child in my class. He had met the author and highly recommended the book. Brandon was an alternative therapy practitioner in the US, who had found a large tumour in her body. She had been medically diagnosed and told that she required surgery. She decided to treat herself and developed a process of deep psychological healing called *The Journey*. She practiced this on herself and cured herself. She speaks of healing at a cellular level and cellular memory in the body, using examples of transplant patients who have had memories from the people who have provided the transplanted organs.

My background is reasonably scientific I have a degree in sports science and geography and I find working at this level of belief too much for me. I know my own mind and if my cancer is a result of something that happened to me in my past using all the negative energy to create cancer in my body, then perhaps it is best left buried. I sure as hell do not want to embark on a process that could be costly and emotionally battering, when I really feel that I need to be positive. I am sure that what I read is true for her, but for me, although very interesting, *The Journey* was a step too far. I learnt a lot and found that she supported the theory of being positive. This I can happily subscribe to.

I then read a book called *Your Life in Your Hands* by Professor Jane Plant. Jane Plant is an earth scientist, a geologist to be precise who was diagnosed with breast cancer. Her book analyses a huge range of research data on cancer, both in the laboratory and clinically with patients. It is hard to absorb the amount of information that she includes and also hard to validate what she says without access to the original data she has assessed. I become quite vocal about some of the research findings she reports, but John, who's a chemical engineer by profession, has to keep reminding me that she is putting her interpretation onto the results she is presenting. I find some of what she writes very interesting, but feel that the way I am approaching my cancer is very different to the way she approached hers. It shows you how unique everyone is.

Professor Plant promotes a change in dietary regime to support good health. This is mostly to reduce the body's inflammatory response, which promotes the growth of cancer cells, and to enhance the immune system, which can help reduce the likelihood of getting cancer in the first place. I wholeheartedly support these two specific recommendations and start to think about how I might change my own diet. She also makes an excellent point about diet and its relationship to cancer. No one is going to make money out of diets, but there is a lot of money to be made out of drugs. So until there are more studies and research into the dietary effects on either contracting or fighting cancer, once you have it then the only research to access is from drug companies and their studies on the efficacy of their drugs; drugs which make them a lot of money. Don't get me wrong, I would not consider stopping the chemo for a second, as the results of such regimens are well documented. I just wonder if in the future we can prevent the increase in cancer in the first place by eating a more simple, healthy diet, much like our parent's generation did.

Finally, the book I find the most useful and the easiest to read is *Anticancer: A New Way of Life* by David Servan-Schreiber. Dr Servan-Schreiber is a French Canadian Neurologist who was diagnosed with a brain tumour, which he discovered by accident whilst having a brain scan for his research when a subject did not turn up for the tests. He looks at very similar information to Professor Plant, but distills the information into four key areas. Two are the same as Professor Plant; diet related to the body's inflammatory response and enhancements to the immune system. He also goes into a lot of detail on both exercise and stress management. I find this book very insprirational and now seriously consider how I should change my diet.

Recuperation

From this I decide to go organic and dairy free; as my cancer is oestrogen receptive, I want to reduce my dietary intake of this hormone. I replace milk with soya milk, which contains phyto-oestrogens. Unfortunately there are mixed views on whether this is better or worse than real oestrogen, but I feel it could not do any harm. There is something to be said about the placebo effect here. If you think that something is going to do you good, it will. Two years further on and I have now replaced this with rice milk.

I now eat some red fruit daily, such as blueberries or raspberries. I rarely drink coffee and regularly drink green tea. My only concern about the dietary changes is that during the winter most of the fruits I want to eat are not in season in the UK, so normally on the packaging I can see how far around the world these items come from. I am not doing much for the environment am I? I have however now switched from Tesco to Waitrose. The range of organic food is so much better and I have now decided that the flavour of organic food is significantly better than non-organic. Is this me justifying my own decision to myself, or is it true? Anyway, I enjoy reading all the books I am given and I find that I learn a lot. It certainly gives me more questions to ask the doctors.

During this time I am in contact with my friend Androulla, who is a homeopath. She has some suggestions for things that I can take to help me manage the potential side effects of the chemo and also to speed my recovery from the surgery. She kindly sends me a set of tiny pills in lots of little plastic sachets, with detailed instructions on what to take for what and when. She won't let me give her any money, so I say I will make a donation for her to my head shaving fund.

Again I am no expert, but before modern medicine came along there were all sorts of things that people took to alleviate illnesses. Yes, I am sure scientists would say it is the placebo effect, but surely there must be something in alternative therapies. I consult with Mary and provide her the list that Androulla has given me, so she can get Dr Fermont to check it out. After all, there is no point in taking something that may clash with the drugs that I am going to be given by the hospital to help me counter the side effects of the chemo.

It is really important to stress here that I am in no way saying I am an expert in my own condition. I have just read lots of books now and made up my own mind as to what I feel is valuable and what will help me. I am still going to accept all the medical treatment that is suggested, as there is a huge body of clinical evidence to support the outcomes that these regimens will produce. The plethora of books about alternative methods of treatment and dealing with cancer can be very confusing, causing possibly some people to opt out of the current treatment available. Don't throw the baby out with the bath water yet, also don't shut your mind to things that you think may help you because if you feel they will, then the psychological benefits of being positive about your condition should only help. I would always let my doctors know what I am doing or thinking, just in case there are any negative side effects that you may not be aware of.

I think this period of reflection helps me come to the conclusion that I want to take control of what I can in relation to the disease and its potential cause. Taking control, but not being obsessive, as this in itself can create stress, is my aim. Changing my diet in this way helps me feel like I am taking control of my body. I am not going to stress over every mouthful of food I take and I am certainly not going to sit and examine every menu at a restaurant, or ask what kind of milk my friends are putting in my tea. But I am going to improve what I put into my body and take control when I can. This really helps me feel that I am personally doing something to reduce the likelihood that the cancer will come back and that can only help me to feel more positive.

Finally, a couple of days before I start chemo, I visit Michael Burke again to get my wound site and scar checked and also to get some fluid drained. After surgery you have drains near the wound site, to drain any blood and serous fluid (the clear fluid you see on top of a graze when it does not bleed). When the drain is removed you can sometimes get a build up of this fluid under the skin. This is called a seroma. I have a small seroma, which Mr Burke drains. He gives me the once over and pronounces me fit to start my chemo. Onward and upwards.

CHAPTER 10

Chemotherapy – Poison that Makes You Better

On 4th December, I need to arrive at the hospital at about tennish and have a blood test. This is so they can see what my blood count and in particular my white cell count is like normally. I will have to have this test every time I have chemo, because if my white cell count is too low, I will be immuno-suppressed and it is too risky to give the treatment.

I get the test done and go upstairs to the chemo suite. This sounds very grandiose, but it is really a room with a desk and space for three large, comfy chairs and a couple for visitors. There are already two other ladies there receiving what I later discover to be herceptin. They have this treatment for a defined period of time after having cancer. This is not something I will need to have.

John has come with me for this first session so that he can see exactly what goes on. Who knows if he will be able to make any of the others with his travel routines? I sit down in the only available treatment chair left and he positions himself to my right. I won't be able to have any needles in that arm, remember.

Mary brings out the tray with all the drugs laid out neatly and goes about getting a cannula into the back of my left hand. The first

Chemotherapy – Poison that Makes You Better

injection through the cannula is an anti-sickness drug. I think back to poor Hunty when he had chemo and how ill he was. Apparently the regimen for testicular cancer is much worse than that for breast, so again I count myself lucky, although of course I was never going to get testicular cancer, was I?

Mary then sets up a saline drip into the cannula, the line of which has a little connecting tap on it for her to attach the syringe that she needs to use to inject the different chemo drugs. The first drug that she starts to inject is bright red. This is the E of FEC, Epirubicin, which is the nastiest of the drugs. If you dropped this on your skin it would burn you, so imagine what it must be doing to the inside of my veins. Mary has to sit patiently and inject it at just the right rate, which she can feel by the pressure on the syringe. She then injects the 5FU, which is colourless. When this is goes in you get a really strange metallic taste in your mouth. Fortunately they kindly provide tea and biscuits to eat, so you don't really taste it. Mary had told me to bring some mints or any other sweet that I fancied, to suck in case I found the taste too horrible. Finally she puts the bag of Cyclophosphamide up when the saline is finished. The whole procedure takes only about an hour and a half, which I don't think is too bad.

Before I leave, Mary gives me a sheet of paper which describes the three different drugs they are giving me, to take home to help counter the side effects of the Chemo. These include Ondansetron, which is the antisickness drug, Dexamethasone, which is a steroid that also helps with the sickness and helps the body repair itself and Zantac, an antacid which helps the stomach manage the ravages of chemo. I will need to take these drugs for three days, which should get me over the worst of the side effects.

John and I leave the hospital and as I am still feeling the benefits of the anti-sickness injection we decide to go shopping in Harrow. There is a 20% off sale in M&S and John needs some new clothes. We have lunch in the café and then do some serious shopping. Retail therapy certainly takes your mind off things and, again, being as normal as possible really helps. I don't want to give in; I had a disease, I am not sick; it is just going to be the treatment that will make me feel sick. I don't want to let it, if I can help it.

Many people carry on work as normal during chemo, in fact I have a colleague at work who worked all the way through her chemo, apart from the days she was actually having it. She was not classroom based however. I have been strongly advised not to teach, partly because the more strain I put on my body, the slower I will recover from each chemo session, also being a primary school teacher means that I will be constantly subjected to all sorts of germs from the children. Why put myself at risk? The other issue is continuity for the children. If I keep having to have time off and then am not well enough to teach, it is really difficult to plan for. Much better that someone is consistently in the class all the time.

That evening I send out my next email update thanking friends for all their support, asking them for no more presents and telling them about the sponsored head shave.

As it turns out, the next day I start to run a temperature. You are given strict instructions that if your temperature goes above thirty-eight degrees centigrade then you need to go straight to the hospital to get checked out. If you are running a fever it could mean that you are neutropenic, which means that your white blood cell count is too low and you cannot fight off an infection. If you have a fever, it could be as a result of being neutropenic, so they need to check by taking your blood. This ends up taking a long time and we spend the best part of four hours that night waiting for the results. Luckily I am not neutropenic, I just have a temperature, which means I am fighting off something.

I consider myself fortunate, as when you think about the list of possible side effects I could experience, I find that I don't suffer too badly. I get a sore mouth only on the first chemo and get somewhat constipated, which is the most uncomfortable thing. My nails definitely deteriorate over time, particularly my toe nails and the veins in my left arm turn much darker and more pronounced. The only long term effect I end up with is the veins hardening and the fat around them being destroyed, so that my left arm looks like it has ridges down it where the veins are. All in all, not as bad as it could have been and definitely not as bad as some people experience. Obviously this excludes hair loss, but that is a different matter.

The next day I start to get into full fundraising mode. John shows me how to set up a fundraising page on Just Giving, which he did when he ran the London Marathon for St Luke's earlier in the year. I create a personal message which describes what has been going on and then include a section which basically just emotionally blackmails people into donating. I know it is shameless, but what harm is there? Why not use my condition to the positive advantage of other people? If I cannot get people to donate now then I am never going to be able to. I send out an email to let everyone know that they can now donate online. This boosts the number of people donating to my Just Giving site and again I get a wonderful assault of emails, making me laugh and keeping me in touch with all my friends.

When I finish the medication to help me through the effects of Chemo, on Sunday, I feel like total shit! Excuse the language, but there is no other way to describe how I feel. I feel way worse than during the chemo, really low, both physically and psychologically. It only lasts for a day or so, but I make a mental note to talk to Mary about it when I next have chemo, to see what she says as to why I may have felt like that. I am sure that with all her experience she will have some light to shed on the situation and some suggestions as to what I can do to counteract these symptoms next time – assuming, of course, that it could happen again.

The following week, I am booked in with Nicky for my first physio session since surgery. You can see how many medical appointments and visits to the hospital I have, so just as well I am not teaching, eh?

Nicky specialises in post-mastecomy care. She carefully assesses my range of movement and is very pleased that I don't seem to be overprotective in the use of that arm and only slightly restricted in how far I can move my right side. She carefully massages the scar and chest area to help break down the scar tissue and shows me what exercises I should be moving onto now. I am keen to go swimming and we discuss it. From a rehabilitation point of view it will be great, but from a germ-catching one during chemo, not so good.

As I am now writing my Christmas cards I feel that it is a good time to tell an even broader community of people about my condition. You must realise that I love people and I am quite good at keeping in touch. It may only be a Christmas card and letter each year, but as email addresses become readily available I have been using that too. I post out approximately 150 cards each year, including family, but I also send over thirty cards to friends who now live abroad – friends from school, university, social groups and work. Then there are the fifty or so which get hand delivered. This doesn't include the children I teach or my colleagues, as I have a practice of making a donation to St Luke's instead.

In preparation to raise as much money as I can, I send out an email to the friends I have not been in contact with recently. This creates a massive spurt of replies from all sorts of people and elicits two very pertinent responses, one who has had testicular cancer and one whose wife has had breast cancer. It just goes to show how prevalent it is.

Whilst all this medical stuff is going on, at school, an opportunity arises. Chris, the head, is doing some work for the local authority (LA) and has funding for one day per week to provide a management development opportunity within the school. He therefore would like to give someone the chance to work as acting deputy head one day per week. Now, even before I qualified, some of my family and close friends have said they thought I would get bored being a teacher and would want to go into management. This is because my career in commerce prior to teaching had me working at senior management level for many years. To some extent they were right, however I love being in class but I just miss the responsibility for adults. Some of this has been covered by the fact that I have some management responsibility already as the continuing professional development leader (CPD), looking after training in the school and having responsibility for initial teacher training (ITT) and newly qualified teachers (NQTs). The chance to work with the head and deputy was a great opportunity to learn the ropes of school management, working at a more strategic level but also experiencing the detailed operational issues that are the bread and butter of day to day life in a school, was a chance I relished.

I express an interest in the job and on 11th December I have an interview with Chris and the chair of governors. They ask me to check with my doctors to make sure that they are happy for me to work one day per week. As it is not classroom based and I will be sitting up in an office at the front of the school, I hope the doctor will say yes. I speak to Mary the chemo sister, who is a little worried and thinks I shouldn't work at all and I also visit the GP, who understands my need to keep myself occupied and have some semblance of normality in my life. I know that Mary is only concerned for my wellbeing and is being very cautious because of all her experience with cancer patients. My need to have something else to focus on other than my treatment is what convinced my GP, who happily signs a sick note that outlines that I can work one day per week, non-classroom based.

I am lucky enough to be offered the position and am really delighted when I get the good news. I will feel connected to the school again and not so cut off. Life in school moves at such a pace that it is really easy to get left behind, however I will not be as out of the loop as if I did not work at all.

My chemo is scheduled for every three weeks, which means that the next time I am due for chemotherapy is Christmas Day. If I had been on the NHS then this probably would not have been an option, but because I am private, amazingly, they actually administer poisonous drugs on bank holidays!

Everyone thinks I am mad to want to have chemotherapy on

I FELT A RIGHT ONE...

Christmas Day, but why not? Disease doesn't stop for public holidays so why delay. I am so keen to keep my treatment on track, every time I defer chemo then it delays the start of the next stage of treatment and that holds up how quickly I can get back to normality. It also does have a financial impact. I get paid full pay for six months and then I drop to half pay, so the longer I am off the longer I will be on half pay.

I am also hoping there is a chance that I will be ready for reconstructive surgery this summer, even though everyone tells me it is highly unlikely. You have to have something to aim for.

CHAPTER 11

Letting My Hair Down or Rather Out!

The weekend before Christmas I am having a shower and washing my hair as normal, when I notice the water isn't draining away. I look down at the plughole and see a huge hair-ball stuck in the plug hole. Oh my goodness, all that hair is from my head. Now I am used to losing quite a bit, as being menopausal I am finding that my hair is falling out anyway. But this is something else. The amount is staggering; at this rate I won't have any hair by Christmas. I find it surprisingly depressing to see such a visibly negative effect of the treatment. Again, I am not in control and I want to be. The minute I am out of the shower and dry I show my sister-in-law, Jo who is visiting with my brother and family, how much hair is coming out.

I get on the phone to Karen, my friend and hairdresser, to see if she can fit me in before Christmas. She says that she can come round on Tuesday night (the day before Christmas Eve). I had planned to have my hair cut after Christmas, as I had been told that the hair starts to fall out between three and four weeks after the first chemo treatment, but there is no way I can just let it fall out at this rate. I'd be looking like a mangy dog in no time.

By the time I actually have my hair cut off I have raised nearly

I FELT A RIGHT ONE...

£2,700, of which well over half has come through Just Giving. People have been so generous – several donations of £100 and one for £1,000, from a trustee colleague at St Luke's. I have already blown my target, so I up it to to £4,000.

Tuesday night Karen comes round to cut my hair. We make an evening of it; we set the kitchen up and get the video camera out and put it on a tripod so the whole thing can be filmed. I have promised the children that they can have a go at cutting some of my hair off. I make sure that we cut a sample off and I put it in a safe place, so that when my hair does grow back I can compare it, to see if it has changed. Apparently people say that the hair comes back thicker or curlier, but definitely different. I want to see if the same thing is going to happen to me.

Lizzie gets the first go with the scissors. Karen counsels her to not cut too close to the scalp as we have not discussed how close to my head she is actually going to cut. Number four, number one? Lizzie hacks away happily, whilst Marcus films and takes photos. Marcus is desperate to have a go to, but does not have too much hair left to play with by the time Lizzie has finished! He has a turn too and tries to create a Mohican. This is difficult to achieve as my hair is so floppy that the bit left in the middle won't stand up and so doesn't really show his handiwork off too well.

Here is a selection of photos from start to finish:

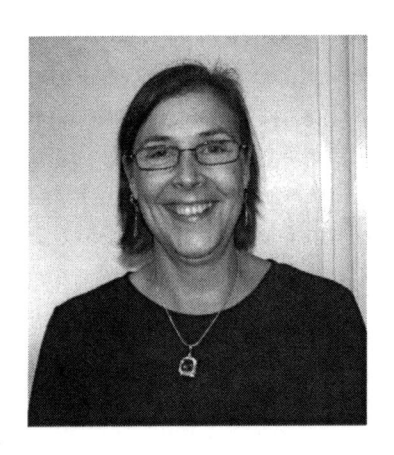

In the beginning!

Letting My Hair Down or Rather Out!

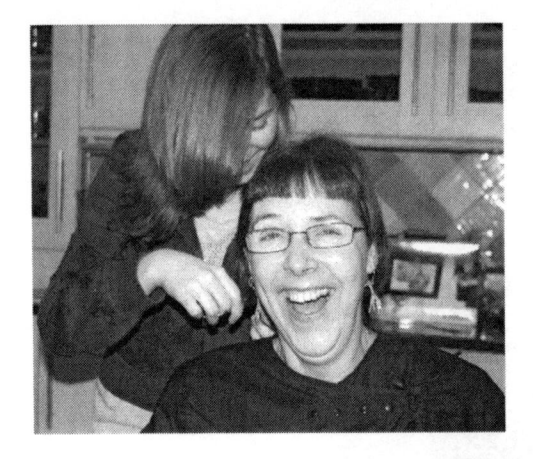

Now that's what I call a mullet!

Okay, let's hand over to a proper hairdresser – Karen, over to you.

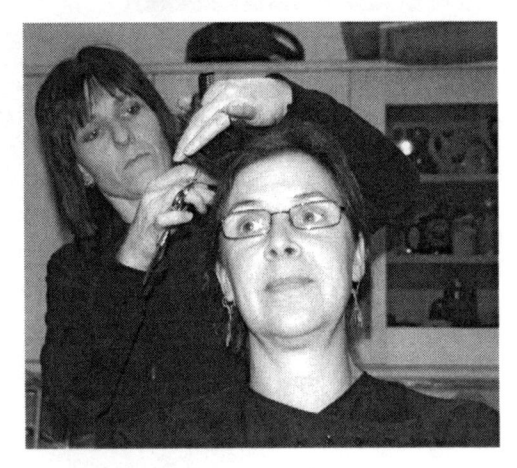

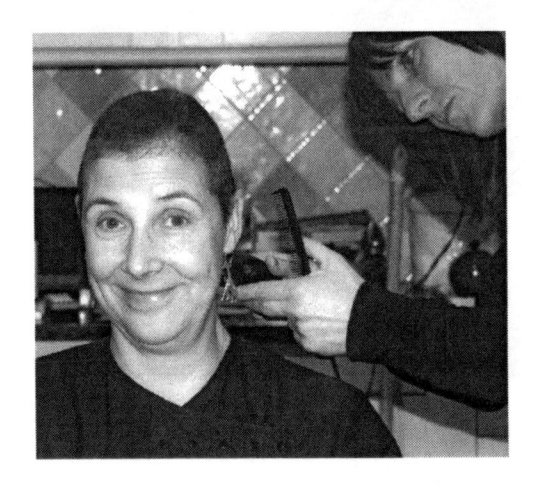

It's getting shorter and now the razor comes out.

I FELT A RIGHT ONE...

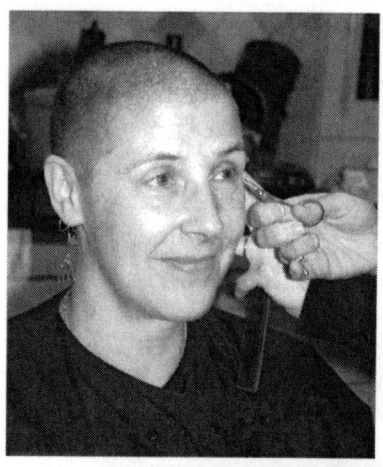

A number one all over, time for a final trim around the ears!

Motey and Johnny look the most alike they ever have and are ever likely to.

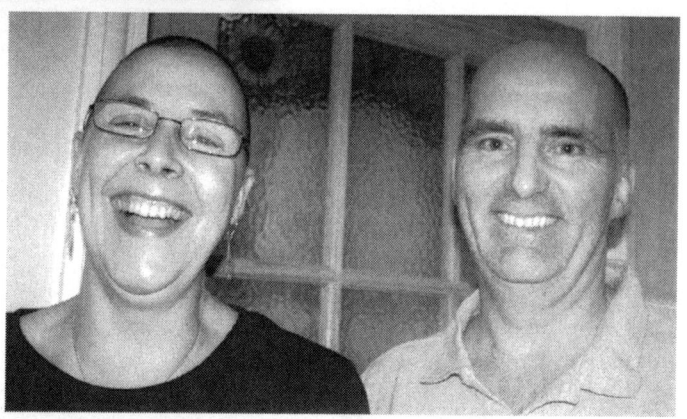

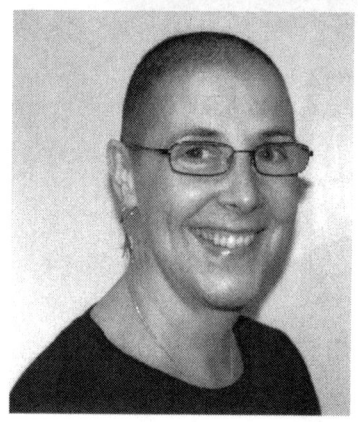

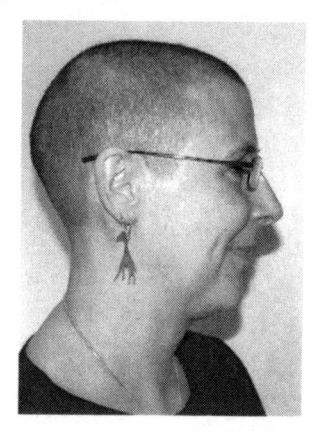

The finished article – not as bad as I thought.

The whole process, although I had been a little worried before, is not nearly as bad as I had thought it would be. Making it a family event and totally involving the children makes it fun. As you can see from the pictures, we laugh quite a lot. The pile of hair on the floor is not as big as I am expecting. I have the whole event captured with moving and still pictures for posterity and also now have the evidence to put up on my Just Giving site, to motivate even more people to donate.

John has his hair done with his usual number one as well. I nearly cried when Marcus offered to have his hair shaved off too. He likes his hair long, so when he told me he was willing to do this, I was very touched. Of course I say no, he doesn't need to do that, but give him a huge hug to show my genuine appreciation of his generous nature.

The email responses are still coming in from lots of people and my friend Gill (the deputy head at school) sends me a short email entitled 'Xmas carols for Christmas day' – The Holly and the I.V. and Chemo ye faithful – I like her sense of humour and it is great to see people making jokes about the situation. I have always been doing it, like when I first tell people I say it is because I thought that 'I should keep them abreast of the situation'.

On Christmas Eve morning, I go and get my blood test done. Later that afternoon I get a call from Mary. I cannot have chemo on Christmas Day as my blood count is too low. I will have to wait till Monday 29th to have another blood test and if that is OK then I can have my second lot of poison.

I am so disappointed, I actually cry. It is the first time I have cried in weeks. I am frustrated. I am not in control and I am really angry about it. In some ways it is a blessing, as it means that we can have a normal Christmas Day and the children won't be too worried about me, but it means a delay, it means I am not on schedule. Is this indicative of things to come? Will my treatment keep getting delayed?

That day I also find out that someone that I know – whose child

I FELT A RIGHT ONE...

I once taught, has just died of pancreatic cancer. He was a real inspiration and had raised so much money through various cycle rides for a charity related to pancreatic cancer. I am truly saddened by this news and again, it makes me realise how lucky I am. The type of cancer I have is not a death sentence, just a hurdle to be overcome. I could have it so much worse.

This evening we had planned to spend with friends. I know I am at risk of catching germs as my white cell count is so low, but I don't want to miss the party and I feel the psychological benefit of socialising is more important than the physical risk of catching something. It is lovely to be out socialising with not too much discussion of my treatment, as most people already know and are in the loop.

Christmas Day is just a really quiet day at home. We wake up not too early, go down to the lounge, sort all the presents out and have a big opening session. The best part for me is always watching the children's' faces as they open the large stocking I have prepared. Lots of little presents, silly things, things that surprise, things that make them laugh. We have a simple lunch at home and then in the afternoon we go for a walk.

On Boxing Day we visit family and generally catch up over the weekend. I cannot go out shopping whilst my blood count is so low because I am so at risk of catching an infection, so I try to avoid large crowds and any friends who have got heavy colds, or who are unwell.

On Monday I go to chemo on my own, as we are expecting my friend Karen and her family (the physio from North Carolina). John stays home waiting for them to arrive.

It is a great relief when Mary tells me that my white blood cell count is good enough for me to have chemo and I settle in for the session. It is exactly the same routine as before and I am done in about and hour and a quarter. Whilst there I discuss with Mary how I felt after the last session, when the effects of the supporting drugs had worn off. She suggests that I might have been 'coming down' from the steroids. As I had not really felt too unwell last time, she suggests I try reducing the dose each day, so that I don't get such a low this time. This I intend to do.

We also discussed the risks of the chemo being postponed again. Mary tells me that if I have two sessions in a row delayed then they would reduce the dose. I ask about how they decide the dose and find out that I am having the maximum. Great! Using my height and weight they calculate skin surface area estimation, which is used to work out the dose.

I have always had a problem with calculations like this. I heartily disagree with the way Body Mass Index (BMI) is used. It is a very crude measure to calculate obesity. It is calculated by dividing your weight in kilograms by your height in metres, squared. It takes no account of bone density and I know I have a large bone structure. I don't wear a size twenty top just for my chest, I also happen to have the shoulders of an East German shot putter! Sorry, I'll get off my hobby horse now, but I do feel qualified to comment on this as half my degree is in sports science.

Anyway, I was not in a position to argue with Mary about the dosage. They know what is best. A good thing about being on the maximum dose is that there should be no chance of missing an errant cancer cell, but can my body cope with this level of poison at each chemo session? Only time will tell. At least I have a reason for the time it is taking my body to recover its white cell count. You know, understanding the factual issues relating to my treatment really does help me to manage the psychological issues that it engenders.

It is great to see Karen and Devin. They live so far away now that I am touched they found the time in their hectic schedule whilst visiting Karen's family in Kent to drive all the way to see us. The children have grown since our visit to them in the US last summer and they quickly make themselves at home. We drink a little! I love the fact that my oncologist says drink 'will not interfere with my treatment at all and so go ahead'. Obviously not getting totally smashed all the time, but a small libation with friends has to be done, in fact it is positively rude not to! John is a staunch red wine drinker and if truth be told is a little bit of a wine snob.

A couple of bottles later and we are all very happy. I realise how much I value so many of my friends; they all seem to have realised that I do want life to be as normal as possible. Yes of course we talk about cancer and my treatment, because they care and they want to know what's going on. However, once covered, we normally move onto other more normal topics of conversation. I do have to remember this and try where possible not to make my condition the focus of the conversation, unless of course I can find an amusing anecdote, which is normally finding a positive spin to lighten the conversation when it gets too heavy.

Karen and family depart the next morning and we as a family get ready to drive down to Wales. We are going to Llandovery for a New Years Eve party. Hunty (the warden – headteacher in other words) is having a big party and as it is a boarding school, all can stay over if they want to. We get to stay in Hunty's house, as being considered the sickest I get top billing. I am really hoping that Hunty's house is warm. One of the possible side effects of chemo, and Hunty told me he also had this problem, is that you get really cold, really easily. I can only assume this is because your capillaries are being frazzled and so are really not up to circulating the blood round your system in the way they normally would. John will tell you that I am like a freezing ice cube in bed anyway. He believes that one of the main reasons I married him is so I can use him as a live hot water bottle. The funniest thing is that being menopausal I am either roasting with a hot flush, or freezing cold like I have sat outside in a snowstorm with no socks and gloves on.

We arrive the day before the party and I have to say that after the three and a half hour journey I am knackered. Hunty comes to the door and gives me the biggest bear hug. He is the first person that I knew really well who had cancer. I know he understands how I feel and what I am going through. His embrace is like a warm blanket enfolding both my body and my heart.

Letting My Hair Down or Rather Out!

That night we go out for a curry in the town, then back to the house to bed. It is minus six degrees outside, very cold indeed and it feels like there is no heating in our bedroom. There is, but it just doesn't feel like it. I go to bed with socks and a beanie hat on! The next day we go out for lunch and then we come home and help Hunty get the library ready for the party tonight. He has all the food prepared and just needs to move a few bookcases and chairs. He has about forty people coming, including staff, family and friends.

The evening is a great success and all Ian's new work colleagues are absolutely lovely. Ian is a saint, he has obviously prewarned people about my baldness. This is the first time that I will be meeting people I don't know whilst bald – quite an interesting experience. Making the decision to be like this does have its negative consequences. Some people do stare, but I am sure only out of curiosity. I am also sure that some people wonder why I would want to display the fact that I have cancer. Part of me feels that it is a badge of honour; I have never felt like wearing a wig, just the thought makes my head itch. What would happen if it slipped, would people look at me strangely? Most of all, why should I have to cover up my condition? It is my choice, I should be allowed to deal with it however I want and basically 'sod' what anyone else thinks. Again I am sure that some people might consider it an attention seeking move, but it has, for me, made me feel totally liberated. Wow, did I ever think in my life I would be totally bald? No. Mind you, I couldn't have chosen a worse time, with one of the coldest winters in decades.

The staring thing is interesting. When we stopped at Leigh Delamare service station on the M4, I did notice people staring. They can't help it. It is not often you see a bald woman in public. For men, of course, it is totally different. John has been doing it for years, so has Hunty, but there is definitely still some level of social inacceptance for a woman to go around without hair. However, staring is an intriguing and sometimes disturbing phenomena.

As a seven year old child, my eldest brother Chris, threw a cup of petrol onto a bonfire (that is what children did in 1956!). The wind blew it back in his face and he went up like a torch. All that was left of the jumper he was wearing was the zip. He spent six months at Mount Vernon Hospital – a specialist burns unit, then back every summer holiday till he was sixteen having skin grafts. He is left today with an inch wide scar which pulls his right ear slightly tight and goes all the way round his chin line to the bottom left hand side of his face. His chest is a mess, mostly scar tissue from skin grafts and the burn itself and a large scar on his right arm.

I was born when Chris was thirteen, so when I was young he would take Justin and me to the cinema or swimming. When we went swimming, I would notice people staring, sometimes open-mouthed, at his scars. It never seemed to bother him, but I was always cross that people could be so rude. Chris couldn't help it, he hadn't burnt himself on purpose to make sure that people looked at him. It was just an accident. This had instilled in me at a very early age a real desire never to do this to someone else. I still work at it today, in fact what I really try to do is to make eye contact, if relevant, and smile at that person. I truly believe, now even more so since becoming a teacher, that staring, particularly at someone who probably doesn't want to be stared at because they have some sort of disfiguring condition or a disability, is damaging to that person's self-esteem. Even if you are not doing so, they may think you are making a value judgement about them which may include pity, misunderstanding, revulsion, even hate. I would never want another human being to think that I thought anything negative about them in terms of what they look, sound, or behave like. I am of course perfectly happy to give killing looks to people who *choose* to behave badly at anytime; this is part of my job as a school teacher!

So, back to being bald – it is enforced on me. It is either that or walk around like an increasingly mangy animal for several months. Yes, I can cover my head in a range of ways, but I don't want to and why should I? So for those people who are staring, I just have to consider that I am forcing this onto them. I could cover up, so it is not really in the same category as my brothers' burn scars. I therefore do try not to resent it, but it is hard. Perhaps it should be more socially acceptable for women to have no hair. Sinead O'Connor did it – but then she is stunningly beautiful. That actress in *Star Trek* did it too, but again she is also a good looking woman.

I find it gives me a great sense of freedom that I have not experienced before in a range of ways; the anti establishment-ist (is there such a word?) in me likes challenging the social norm; the marketeer in me likes the opportunity to raise awareness of cancer and its effects; the self-consciousness in me finds it makes me feel less self-conscious. I will never worry about what my hair looks like again in any major way. If a haircut goes wrong I know it will grow back and no-one is going to stare at me nearly as much as they do now.

After a great party and a lovely couple of days with good friends, it is time to return home.

CHAPTER 12

Just When You Think it is All Going So Well

On Monday 5th January it is a training day and we are working on coaching and mentoring for the whole school staff. This is something dear to my heart and I hope is a good day for all. Then the very next day is my first official day as 'acting deputy head'. It is so great to be in school and feeling an element of normality creep slowly back into my life.

When I am not in school I try to keep myself busy. This is with a mixture of things; coffee (well, tea for me) with friends, reading, a bit of sleeping if I feel really tired, (although I do try to avoid this as I then find it very difficult to get to sleep properly at night) and some work bits that I can do on the PC at home.

I start writing a story about my journey, which I will later use as the focus for this book. I discover computer games and also do a little on the Wii Fit that I was given for my birthday. The one thing I do not get into is watching daytime TV, I feel this would be a slippery slope for me and, truly, when I was in hospital I discovered that there was not that much I was interested to watch. I am more a movies person, which I don't like doing on my own, so there is very little TV during the day.

Just When You Think it is All Going So Well

I am generally just getting on with life and getting through the chemo, which isn't as bad as I thought it was going to be. However, I am starting to get really bad back pain now. A little bit of history here – I was diagnosed with arthritis of the spine when I was thirty and have had a disk removed from my neck between the C5 and C6 vertebrae, because I started to lose the feeling in my thumb and forefinger. This was back in 1997 when Lizzie was eleven months old. I am really careful with my back and sleep with an orthopaedic pillow, which goes everywhere with me if an overnight stay is required, I also never sleep on my front. John has got used to the extra pillow I use either under or between my knees, depending if I am laying on my back or side. When I was pregnant it was even worse: there was barely any room left in the bed for him with extra large me and my collection of pillows.

The pain makes it hard to go to sleep at night and it is steadily getting worse. I arrange to see my friendly osteopath Tony and he checks me out and treats my lower back to sort out the pain. It does feel slightly better and I drive home. At night now the pain is so bad that I have to go down and lay on my back on the lounge floor with my legs bent resting on a stool or coffee table. Tony suggested I do this and it does relieve the pain for a while, but makes it impossible to sleep. I also resort to having hot baths in the middle of the night, as well as one before bed, again this helps, but the pain still gets worse. I am by now getting almost no sleep at all. I am working on the Wednesday in school, my second day in my new temporary job. It keeps my mind busy and helps with the pain. I am exhausted with so little sleep, but I still enjoy being in school. There is no way I would have managed teaching in class.

On Friday I have an appointment at Northwick Park to have my proper silicone prosthesis fitted. I visit the breast care department, where the specialist nurses relating to all aspects of breast cancer are based. This is where I had gone to talk through getting breast cancer and to have my arm measured before my mastectomy.

Anna is lovely and looks carefully at the shape of my remaining breast to see which brand and type of prosthesis will suit me best. She chooses a couple for me to try and we find one that is perfect. It is slightly asymmetrical and is definitely a 'right' one. Some come in a shape that can be used bilaterally, but the shape of my breast demands one that that is unilateral. The only negative is that I will not be able to wear an underwired bra with this prosthesis, as it goes slightly round the side of my chest and the wire would dig in possibly damaging the silicone and making it leak. I have come wearing a close fitting shirt so that it is easy to check if the prosthesis looks OK. I am really pleased with the result and truly believe that if you did not know I'd had a mastectomy then you would never know the difference. I just have to be careful not to wear too plunging or loose tops, so that the concave part of my upper chest is not too visible, also so that you cannot see down the top when I lean over as it would then be very apparent something was amiss down there. I go home to sort out my wardrobe and put away what I can't really wear for a while.

I also take a visit to Nicola Jane, a shop in Farringdon that specialises in all things mastectomy related, including underwear, modesty panels, swimsuits, prostheses and other paraphernalia. I buy a swimsuit, some special bras with a pocket in to hold my new prosthesis and a specialist swimming prosthesis. This one is made of chlorine resistant, translucent, colourless silicone. It has special drainage channels at the back to let the water flow through and out as you swim. I feel it looks a little like a jelly fish, but I am not complaining. No one is going to see it except me and the family and if it means I can get exercising then I am happy.

I actually try swimming for the first time with my new prosthesis. I don't get changed in the main section, but in one of the small cubicles. I am a little concerned at how I might frighten small children with the way my body looks at the moment. I am hoping that the exercise will ease the pain in my back and leg, by helping loosen everything up. It doesn't hurt to swim any more than normal and it really helps my chest. I can feel it making it easier to stretch and working the arm muscles feels really good. I swim about sixteen lengths because if I do the Hatch End Triathlon, this is the distance I will have to be aiming for.

By Saturday night I have now had the back pain for the best part of ten days, with it gradually increasing in severity – a pain that is deeply in my right buttock and all the way down my right leg. Very like sciatica, which is what I am convinced it is. I just think that my pain threshold is reduced by the chemo. In the end, after a totally sleepless night crying and at my wits end, John takes me to Northwick Park Hospital A&E department. It is about 6.00am on Sunday morning. We leave a note for the children in case they wake up, but hope we will be back before they do. I really don't want to bother anyone at that time of the morning and we should only be gone an hour or so.

6.00am on a Sunday morning is a good time to visit an A&E department, if that is what you have to do. It is virtually empty. I register at the reception desk, tell them I am on chemo and I am truly impressed at how quickly they see me. I feel like sick royalty, I am seen by a triage nurse so quickly. I am in so much pain; I cannot sit down and instead stand rocking backwards and forwards. John starts to giggle to himself. I look at him quizzically.

"You know the only difference between you and a Romanian orphan is that you're not chained to the bed," he chirps, trying to cheer me up.

I am in so much pain that I don't really see the funny side just then. Well I do, but not enough to register a laugh. Within minutes the doctor comes to see me and sends me immediately for an x-ray. Again, within only minutes the radiologist takes me through to sort me out. She can see I am in agony and is incredibly gentle with me. We get chatting, as even though I am in pain my normal social side comes to the fore. We discover someone in common as if often the case: a colleague of hers is the father of a boy I teach at school. She is speedy and sends me back to the doctor incredibly quickly. Soon the doctor returns and shows me the x-ray on screen. There is definitely something amiss between two of my lumbar vertebrae, L4 and 5. The bones at the end of each vertebra appear to be a noticeably different colour than they should be and stick out like a sore thumb, or sore back as it actually is, on the x-ray.

He tells me that I need to go back to the doctors treating me and get a more detailed assessment done on my back, but he thinks this may be the cause of the pain. He already has in his hand a pack of Temazepam, which he had noticed was the last pack in the drugs cupboard. He reckoned I needed it very badly so had kept it aside especially for me. Now that is really thoughtful. I go home, take a tablet and finally get a couple of hours sleep. All in all, the whole visit took just under an hour. Pretty darn good.

The next day is my next chemo session. I go to the hospital at 9.30 to get my regular blood test done and fantastically everything is fine. Yippee! No time lost this time. Zoe has come with me as my chemo buddy for this treatment and it will give her a chance to catch up with Mary, as they used to work together. It is nice to have company during the treatment as it takes your mind off what is actually happening to your body. The steroids they give to help you through the chemo also work like magic on my back. I had never thought I would ever be grateful for chemo, but I truly am. The medication helps me get the best night's sleep in weeks – still fitful, but certainly a few hours. The restorative value of sleep can, in my mind, never be underestimated.

During my chemo visit, I talk to Mary about the situation and she immediately phones my oncologist David Fermont who arranges an urgent referral to Sean Malloy, an orthopaedic surgeon specialising in backs. They also get me sorted for an emergency MRI scan to be done that Thursday. What I don't realise at the time, but discover later, is that the urgency is because they are all concerned about the cancer having spread to the bone in my spine. I am quite glad I don't realise this then.

That afternoon I make a visit to the Harrow Teacher's Centre to make a presentation. I feel so normal on the supporting drugs.

Again, keeping busy and exercising my mind really helps. They very sweetly present me with a bunch of flowers and I tootle off home to have a rest.

I keep very busy this week as the busier I am, the less pain I seem to feel. My friend Dave, who I was at university with, brings his nine month old who I have not yet met over for tea. I have lunch at a company I used to work at in Chertsey, to visit a colleague who is visiting from Cape Town.

Thursday's MRI comes round quickly, but nothing will be forthcoming until the radiologist (the doctor who will analyse the scans and make a diagnosis) reports back to the surgeon. I just need to wait and see.

Whilst sitting watching TV with John over the weekend I feel a really hot, itching sensation at the top of my right leg and in the groin area. I take off my trousers and notice a patchy, bright red rash near my groin. I also notice some spots near my knee and at the bottom of my right ankle. I say to John I had better make an appointment with the GP tomorrow as it slowly dawns on me. Has all this pain been shingles all along?

First thing in the morning I call the GP and I go in that afternoon. Yep, it is shingles. Why hadn't it occurred to me before? There had been no rash. All this pain is nerve pain. The doctor prescribes Aciclovir (an antiviral) and Amitriptyline (something to help the nerve pain). She also prescribes some Diazepam to help me sleep until the pain recedes. What a huge relief to know what it is and that it can actually be treated. Within hours of taking the medication I start to feel a lot less pain and it is amazing. Really good sleep also helps. I stop taking the sleeping tablets at the same time as I finish the other medication. I do not want to become reliant on them for sleep. I have to miss going into school this week, until the rash scabs over, as I could be contagious to any people who have not had chickenpox. Unlikely, but the doctor tells me I should stay home.

John is away in Germany this week and I have arranged for Zoe to come with me to see Sean Malloy, the orthopaedic surgeon to get the scan results. I tell him that I have shingles, just in case he has not had chickenpox, as if he hadn't he could possibly catch it, especially if he was going to touch my skin during the examination.

He thanks me, but says he is fine. He gives me the physical once over and recognises the tell tale signs of the shingles following a nerve path down my right leg. He comments that it is an unusual place to get it, as most often it is found on the abdomen.

After the examination and parallel pleasantries I sit back down at his desk. He looks me straight in the eye and says, "Well you'll be pleased to know that there is no spread of the cancer to your spine!"

I hadn't really considered this a possibility. If I had thought about it; I had definitely pushed it to the back of my mind, and so was a little taken aback. I look at Zoe and she comments, "Well I had thought about it, but didn't want to worry you."

Ignorance on this occasion was definitely bliss. Or is it that I just don't really consider the negative possibilities associated with this disease? It doesn't really matter, because at least I hadn't been worried sick and neither had John.

Sean goes on to talk about the fact that I have a missing disk between the two lumbar vertebrae L4 and L5. The area that had shown up on the x-ray at A&E was the wear and tear showing on the bone as a result, whilst he also comments there is a small tear to the disk lower down between L5 and the sacrum (the five fused vertebrae between your lumbar spine and your coccyx, or tail bone). I say that it is remarkably careless of me to have lost a disc and not even know about it. Sean asks me if I remember a time of significant back pain in the past and I can think of two occasions where I ended up flat on my back for a few days: once when I was twenty one and once whilst carrying a heavy backpack round the world in Bali, 1989. It could have been on either occasion.

I ask if there is anything that I should not be doing, as I am keen to get running again, with every intention of entering the Hatch End Triathlon this year. He really appreciates the fact that I need to do something physical, even though it may not be the best thing for my body. He does suggest that I should not run any more, but that if I really feel I want to then to go ahead and if I have problems, to come back and he will sort me out. He says that if, when the shingles has settled, I am still in any pain then to come back and see him. I really warm to Sean as both a doctor and person. He is pragmatic and obviously understands what drives me. Not all doctors, especially surgeons, are like this, and I recognise a very special person when I meet one.

On the way home, I thank Zoe for coming with me. I am really glad she came. Sometimes when you meet the doctors it helps to have someone else hear what you hear, just in case you interpret it wrongly. She is so relieved that the cancer had not spread and I feel sorry that I unknowingly put her through this worry. That's the problem with people in the medical profession, I sometimes think they know too much and this can make them worry more than your average person like you and I. So, truly, ignorance can be bliss.

I do more social catching up at the end of the week, when the scabs have formed, as with the drugs keeping all the pain at bay, I feel like I am firing on all cylinders again.

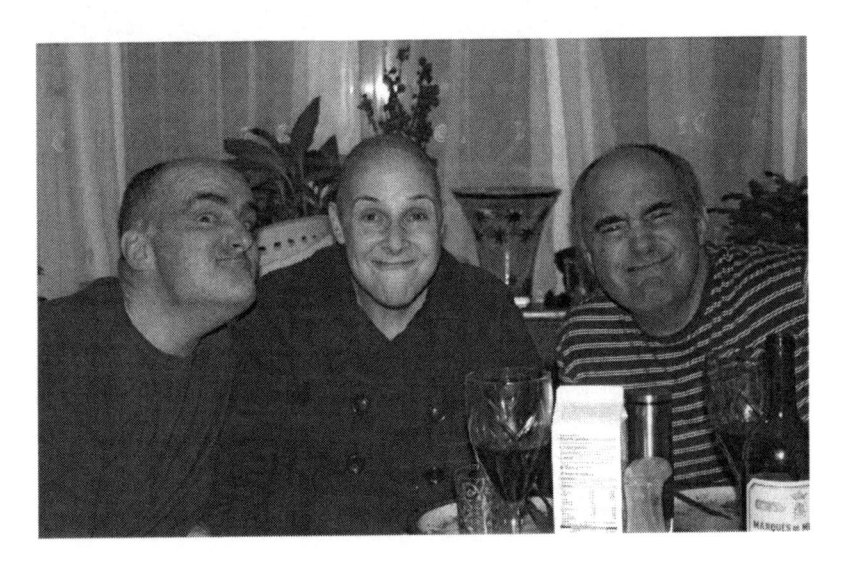

I FELT A RIGHT ONE...

Monday morning dawns to eight or so inches of snow outside. I have had a message from Lizzie's school that it is closed and I am pretty sure that my school will be too. Even though I am not due to work today day, I have a feeling they will need all the help they can get staffing the phones and helping sort things out. I don my very bright 1980's ski suit, put on my boots, gloves and hat and walk up to school. There are several people in, but it is all hands on deck.

On returning home, I find my children have been in the street with all the other children in the local area and have made massive snowmen. I help and we even make a snow dog. With time on my hands that Monday, I send out another update to the enlarged list of email contacts. I let them know that I have reached my target of £4,000.

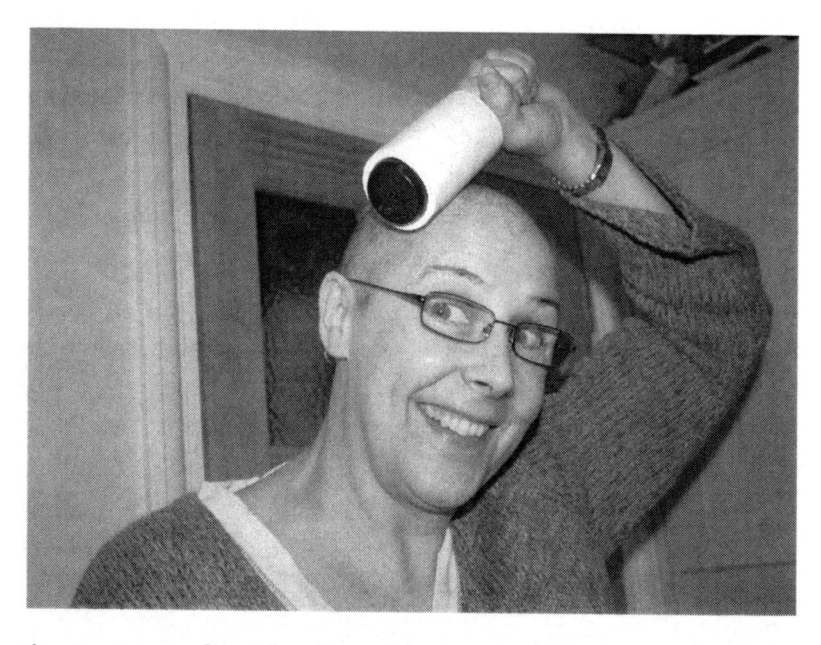

As you can see from the photo, I have resorted to brushing my hair with an anti-fluff roller. I also find I have to do this to my pillow and my clothes. I basically have hairy dandruff and the only way to deal with it is meet it head on, sorry about the pun. Each morning I roll my head and make sure all the loose hair is removed so that I don't shed as much during the day. I know I make myself sound like some sort of moulting animal, but that is actually what it is like. I have to get Karen back a couple of times to give me a 'number one' again, as the hair that has not actually fallen out, which is not much, does still keep growing.

The next day I am supposed to be in school, but it is shut on the advice of the local authority. By then most of the snow has melted on the roads. It really didn't last too long. I am glad to see that my snow angel has survived for the moment. I have another busy week, with a conference at the teacher's centre, a visit to Tony (my osteopath) and a fundraising meeting at St Luke's. At the fundraising meeting they all tell me they are not surprised at how well my sponsorship for the head shave is going. The total is at £4,355 at the moment.

I also have a check up with the optician to discover what effects the chemo is having on my eyesight. I had thought I was not seeing too well and it is confirmed when the ophthalmologist says my eyes have deteriorated by one diopter. This is quite a lot in a short space of time. He tells me not to worry, that this is a standard problem during chemo and that my eyes will return to normal a few months after I finish. He was spot on and they are now absolutely fine.

On Monday, believe it or not, it is chemo day again. It does come around so quickly and I am sure it is because I keep myself busy. I go for my blood test at 9.30 and by 10.30 I am ready to come home, as yet again my blood count is too low. At least this time I am not so down about it. Yes, I am frustrated, but why worry about what you cannot change. Having dealt with it once before, I know I can deal with it again. I am booked in for Thursday lunchtime.

Again a busy week, work-wise, I have a meeting at the teachers centre and a live coaching practice session (based on the course I attended last October) at a local high school. Thursday comes round quickly and I go for my blood test at 11.30am. By 12.30 I am having chemo again. By now the veins in my left arm are starting to turn an interesting colour and they have become really tight. They call it 'cording'. Some of the fat around the veins gets destroyed and when I compare my arms to look at, you can definitely see that something is amiss. This is of course a normal side effect of chemo and you just have to live with it. The arm does get sore and wearing a watch can sometimes be uncomfortable. I am now in the habit of taking my watch off at night time, which definitely helps. I go to this session on my own, as it is difficult to plan things when your appointments keep getting delayed, so I have decided that even though people have kindly offered to be my chemo buddy I may be best going by myself.

For some reason, this fourth chemo session really knocks me for six. I am exhausted and actually have to rest significantly over the weekend. It is not that I feel sick, but more like I feel I have been run over by a steam roller. It is frustrating to feel so crap, when I felt I had been managing the chemo so well. Every little small change in how you feel can feel like a setback and I don't want to let my thoughts turn to the negative. Zoe and Mary have both told me that as you go through chemo there is a cumulative effect and that towards the end each bout affects you more, so that must be the reason. At least John is around at the weekend, which is great as we are having a small party to celebrate Lizzie becoming a teenager

It is also about this time that a colleague at work also discovers she has breast cancer. She has to have a mastectomy, but blessedly does not have to have chemo or radiotherapy. It makes me really think about things. I am worried that because of the way I have handled my cancer at school and been so open, she might feel she has to handle herself in a certain way. I have learnt that every individual deals with cancer differently and you cannot impose your way on anyone else. However, other people looking at us may expect us to behave in a similar way, because we have the same disease. That would be unfair. We talk on the phone and agree to meet up when she is feeling up to it.

As I still find that I have some time on my hands, I decide I need a project to keep me occupied. I decide it is time to build a den at the bottom of the garden. Both Lizzie and Marcus play the drums and at the moment their drum kit is in the loft bedroom, taking up a lot of space. I am also really conscious of the amount of noise the children make for the neighbours who have young children, so I don't let them play after 6.30 which is a bit restrictive. I also feel that as the children are becoming older they would like a space of their own, where they can take their friends when they come round. I also think that when they grow up, I can turn it into an exercise room or office. I start to draw up plans and get some quotes from builders.

Another benefit of having cancer is that I had a critical illness policy which I took out when I was working at Orange. I had made a claim and they had paid up. The money will be put aside for the long term, in case my prognosis gets worse. After all, that is what it is for. However, I do feel I can spend some! You know money is there to spend. Eamonn says the last cheque you write before you die should bounce! The only problem is, none of us actually know when this will really happen and of course I wouldn't want to run out, but I like the sentiment.

My social life is still on the up and up and I meet up with two really old friends, who I used to work with at Comparex in 1990, who got in touch before Christmas. To me, this has been such a wonderfully positive side effect of getting cancer. I am really enjoying having the time catching up with all these friends who have made such an effort to get back in contact with me

February 13th is Lizzie's thirteenth birthday and on Sunday she is having a party – just a few friends to go bowling and have pizza. I know that some of her friends know about me being sick, but I have checked with her to make sure that she tells all her friends who are coming why I am bald. I am concerned that they might be embarrassed if they don't know and I feel it is only fair that they have been told before they arrive. I have the impression that Lizzie doesn't really like telling people or talking about it, but she does tell them before they come and that puts me much more at ease. It

I FELT A RIGHT ONE...

seems they all have a lovely time and it is a great start to the half term week, where we also head down to Brighton for a few days.

The next week I again have visitors who I used to work with at Orange. We haven't seen each other for about five years and it is as if we had only seen each other yesterday. It makes me realise that the reason we can't fit in seeing all our friends is that when you have children, their activities seem to take up all your time. As my children are starting to get older now, it is getting slightly easier.

The start of March brings with it another hectic week. The builders are starting on the den at the bottom of the garden and again it is really nice to have something else to keep me occupied. I keep the workforce fed and watered with tea/coffee and biscuits.

I also start running, only a few times and only a mile or so. My legs feel like lead and my lungs seem not to be able to process the air quickly enough to feed my body, but the effects afterwards are amazing. Not physically, but mentally. In fact, it may not have been the best thing to do for my body, as surely I am putting it under enough strain with the chemo, but I had asked the doctors and they had said if I felt like I could, then I was welcome to try. So I try and am glad I do. It makes me feel great, as I say, the mental buzz it gives me more than makes up for the fairly significant physical discomfort! I really feel like I have achieved something each time I run and that positive boost to my self-esteem and confidence is brilliant.

Negativity for me is worse than the chemo, as it poisons my mind, which in turn poisons my body. If you think you can't do something then you are never going to achieve it. This continual craving for normality just keeps pushing me to do things that surprise me and sometimes worry other people, but if I let the chemo get to me any more than it needs to then I would be silly. Luck is on my side in terms of how sick I feel after each session. The drugs, the homeopathic remedies and my bloody mindedness help me in addition to my body's lack of a massive negative response to the actual chemotherapy. I am so blessed.

I am working on Tuesday and then on Wednesday I meet a

Just When You Think it is All Going So Well

friend for lunch. That afternoon I go back to see Michael Burke for my check up. He is pleased with my progress and I use this opportunity to talk about breast reconstruction. We talk through the choices and I explain that my preferred option is the free perforator flap, as it is the only method I have researched that does not require any foreign items to be placed in your body afterwards. Michael does not do this kind of reconstruction himself and recommends me to a plastic surgeon called Adam Searle, who works from the Royal Marsden Hospital. I ask if he will make a referral for me, which he does. He carefully prepares me for the fact that my timescales of wanting the surgery this year are really a bit optimistic. He feels that I would have to wait for at least three months after radiotherapy, which at this rate won't happen till May. This would mean taking time off at the beginning of a new academic year. Not a good idea. He also suggests that I might want to give my body more time to recover from the ravages of the chemo and radio, and I should consider taking time to get fit again, ready to handle an even more major surgery than my original mastectomy.

That night my friend Simone comes round for dinner. I tell her all about what Michael Burke has said and she tells me that she is really glad he is managing my expectations. She definitely wants me to wait till next year to have the surgery, so that I give myself time to recover. Again I don't like being told 'no', but I am beginning to realise that it is only because my friends care for me and want me to do the right thing.

I think the reason I want to get the reconstruction over and done with as soon as possible is so that I feel I am finished with everything and totally back to normal. Waiting for the reconstruction will feel like I am on hold, in limbo. It is a really major operation and will take a large amount of time to recover, so realistically it may be better to wait till next summer (2010), take the last few weeks of term off and use the summer holidays as part of my recuperation.

The next day is chemo day and again it has come round so quickly. I arrive at 9.30, have my bloods taken and patiently wait until Mary tells me the results. Guess what, it is a no go. My blood count is too low, yet again. Mind you, I am not really surprised as I had felt so tired and low after the last one. Oh well, I guess it is a lesson in patience for me, a lesson I definitely need to learn. We arrange a time for next Tuesday and also book in a visit with David Fermont.

That day I am also due to visit Xenia, my colleague who has recently had her mastectomy. I go over for lunch and it is really good to spend time with her. Being able to talk to someone about what you have gone through and are going through is a very cathartic experience. Sharing the silly things that annoy you, which no one else would really care about, is quite reassuring and I feel we both greatly benefit from the time spent together. Xenia has the added worry that she is the second person in her family to have breast cancer; her sister had it only last year. What kind of luck for two sisters to be struck down with the same cancer within such a short period of time?

By Friday the builders are ready to pour all the foundations for the den, several tonnes of it in fact. A large cement mixer arrives and they feed a pipe all the way through the house (the hall and kitchen) down to the bottom of the garden to pump the concrete. I am a little nervous in case the pipe bursts or a joint breaks and tonnes of concrete line the inside of my house. Not a nice thought! I walk down to a neighbour's house for a cup of tea until it is all over.

John is away quite a lot at the moment, this coming week he is in Russia and two weeks later, Egypt. I know he doesn't really like travelling, especially when I am due for chemo, but what can he do? It is his job. I know he is a lot more relaxed now that he knows I am not suffering too badly through the treatment and he is also reassured by how much support I am getting. It makes it easier for him in this quite difficult situation.

CHAPTER 13

A Light at the End of the Tunnel Gets Darker before Getting Lighter Again

The following Monday I am working in school and then Tuesday is my rescheduled chemo session. I arrive for blood tests at 11.00am and am very relieved when given the all clear for treatment. This is the fifth one, so after today only one more to go. I think I can see the light at the end of the tunnel. I have my treatment and towards the end of the session David Fermont arrives and, as there is no one else in the chemo suite, he joins me and we sit and chat. We talk through what will happen at the end of chemotherapy, about how long I will need to wait before I start radiotherapy and when I will start taking the Tamoxifen. I ask a question that I have wanted to know the answer to for quite a while, but have not had the opportunity to ask.

After the operation, the chemo, the radio and taking Tamoxifen for five years, what is the percentage likelihood that I will get a recurrence of the cancer? He starts off by saying if I had only had the operation and no other treatment, there would still have been a 20%, which is a one in five chance, of getting the cancer again. Then

I FELT A RIGHT ONE...

he goes on to explain that by having all the additional treatments and therapies I have now reduced that rate to 10%. Still a one in ten chance of it coming back! I am shocked. I don't think I show it. I don't really know what I was expecting, but it wasn't this, so perhaps I did have an idea and just didn't like the fact that his idea didn't match up to my wishful thinking. I think I had in my mind that it would be as low as 5%. A one in twenty chance sounds so much less than a one in ten.

I leave the meeting after treatment and as I am walking out, I bump into Elaine, the breast care nurse. She asks me how it is going and I burst into tears. She finds an empty office, takes me in and sits me down. She encourages me to talk about how I am feeling. I explain that I am shocked by what David has just told me. In fact, I realise I am actually angry and frustrated. All this crap treatment, this poison, the nausea, the shingles, the permanent exhaustion, the total disruption of my life and all for just an extra bloody 10%. I know that sounds ungrateful and silly, but that is what it feels like to me. I am processing my feelings on the hoof and poor Elaine is bearing the brunt of it. It really helps to let it all out though. I definitely believe that bottling up ones emotions is not a good thing and that getting it all out as quickly as possible means you can move on more quickly, well for me anyway. I feel better having spent the time with Elaine and I am really grateful to have bumped into her.

I go home feeling better, but very flat. John is away and I could really do with talking it through with him. He always has something valuable to contribute to my thought processes and often sheds a different perspective on things that I may not have considered. It is times like this that I hate the fact he is away. When we speak on the phone that evening, I can tell he is just as fed up as I am, because he cannot be there to make me laugh and cheer me up.

I guess I had this coming really. I had been so upbeat for so long and had not really had a cry since Christmas Eve, when I knew I was not going to have chemo on Christmas Day. Ten weeks without a melt-down is pretty good really, but I don't like being down. The only good thing is I know I will bounce back up again and having been down you appreciate the 'feeling good' times even more. It is rare to see me this low and the kids are great. They can see when I need a hug and they take it in turns to sit next to me and give me a cuddle. This makes me feel even worse! I don't want them to get upset, just because I am. When you are feeling terrible it just takes that one person to ask if you are OK and you would have been if only they hadn't asked… The children recognising my need and giving me comfort just makes me even more emotional and I am a weepy mess for the rest of the evening.

On Thursday I catch the train to Tring to have lunch with Carol. I am still a bit of a mess really; better, but not back to my normal positive self. Carol is brilliant, an ex nurse, reiki master, ordained interfaith minister and bereavement specialist. She knows just what to say and doesn't actually try to make me feel better, rather just lets me work my way through it myself by talking about it. I don't think she realises what a skilled and gifted listener she is. I have a lot to learn from her.

Meanwhile, the building work is coming on a treat and the walls are nearly complete. It is looking a bit of a monstrosity at the moment and I know our neighbours at the back are a little concerned. However, I know that I don't want to look at something horrid and have decided on a pitched rather than flat roof. When Bobby tells them this, their mind is put at rest.

On Friday I have a meeting at St Luke's and then in the evening dinner with friends, the same group who got together just before I had my surgery. These guys always make me laugh and, truly, laughter is the best medicine. After a really low week, I feel I have regained my sense of perspective and that I am back to my normal, positive self again.

The next week I am quite tired so, I don't do too much. I swim again, which although tiring boosts my energy levels and acts like physiotherapy for my arm and chest. When I saw Michael Burke the other week I had talked about the strange sensation you feel

I FELT A RIGHT ONE...

under your arm. This is because a nerve gets cut when they remove the lymph nodes you lose a large part of the feeling in the skin in your armpit and down the inside and back of your arm. He described it as feeling like you are carrying a grapefruit round under your arm and he was right. I would describe mine more as feeling like a satsuma, so I am obviously lucky as they are definitely smaller than grapefruits! The only problem he had ever encountered with a patient because of this was that she had made a hot water bottle too hot and burnt her skin in her armpit because she couldn't feel it. As I use Johnny as my hot water bottle and he won't fit under my armpit, I should be alright!

My very local friends come around again this week to keep me company. I work on Friday and then in the evening go up to Carol's house for a Temple Spa party, where her friend Yvette is showing a range of skin treatments and body care products. I have a lovely evening and get chatting to Carol's mum, Gill, who had breast cancer over fifteen years ago, which was really reassuring. To see living proof that people do come through breast cancer perfectly fine is great. I know I am going to be fine and have always been confident about this, but it does no harm to meet and talk to people who have had similar experiences which reinforce this view.

The next week, whilst at work, I try wearing some of the headgear I have been bought. There is one really pretty Harley Davidson headscarf with diamantés on it which Brian had given me whilst in Dubai last year. By the end of the day the indentations on my forehead when I take if off make me look like Vivien out of the *Young Ones* with stars stuck on my forehead! I will only wear that one for short periods of time in the future.

This week is busy with a visit from Hunty, a shopping trip to Biscester Outlet Village with Sarah, a catch up with a colleague from work, a day in school, a St Luke's board meeting and most importantly my first visit to see the plastic surgeon, Adam Searle. Carol had kindly said that she would come with me, but John's travel plans changed and he is actually able to join me. Carol would have been fantastic, but I am really glad that John is there as I want him to be part of the whole process. He needs to know what I am letting myself in for, as he will have to be the one who supports me through it.

We meet Adam at his clinic in Central London and again I am struck by what a delightful person he is. I think that for the primary surgeon like Michael Burke who has to be the person to deal with all the negative side of the illness such as removing the cancer, giving the results of the test and giving the basic prognosis, it must be very wearing over time and is possibly a more difficult job psychologically. Not that Michael ever showed this, he was always charming, kind and positive.

The plastic surgeon, though, is helping you through the next stage, which is getting your body back to as normal a state as possible and is, therefore, automatically more positive. Both surgeons are of course remarkably skilled and amazing people. I find the whole experience of discussing how we can get my body back to a more normal shape really exciting.

He takes us through each type of reconstruction and what it means. I have already done my homework and tell him that my preference is for a free perforator flap. He asks why and I go through my reasons: I don't want any silicone implants; I don't want to have to have mesh in my stomach to stop future herniation after they have used the muscle; and I don't want to use fat from a part of my body, like my bottom, which would then mean that I would not really have a symmetrical bum! I would like all the fat taken from my tummy (of which there is plenty) and have it used to reconstruct my chest. No foreign objects and I get a tummy tuck into the bargain.

He tells me I am doing the right thing by thinking so far ahead and that Michael Burke has done well in managing my expectations. Adam would not even consider looking at me till at least September and possibly longer, depending on how my skin and tissue in my chest recover from radiotherapy.

He agrees that as I have a rather large chest, a reduction of my remaining left one and transplanting the skin, fat and associated blood vessels from my stomach to create a new right breast would definitely give me the best outcome. He tells me that being in a fairly physical job, I should allow twelve weeks for a full recovery, which definitely means I need to wait till summer 2010. Of course I could have it done sooner, but I really don't want to take extended time off in the middle of an academic year. I don't believe it is fair on the children and it would be incredibly disruptive.

I have a full list of questions to ask him, one of which is how many times he has performed this operation and how many times it has failed. I have looked up the general statistics and about 5% is the average failure rate for this type of surgery; the most common failure being in the reconnection of the transplanted arteries and veins. As you can imagine, if the blood supply fails then the tissue dies and that is that. He tells me that he has successfully performed this surgery over 200 times and in all his time on this particular type of operation, he has only twice had a problem where the vascular transplantation has not worked. So his failure rate is less than 1% which, to my mind, sounds good. I am very pleased with my choice of surgeon, or rather the one who was recommended to me!

I ask if I should grow some more fat on my stomach to make sure I have enough to make a large enough breast, but he tells me not to worry, he would rather I didn't put on too much weight as it is better to be lighter and healthier than worry about the size chest I am going to end up with. We agree that I should come back later this year or early next year, to talk in more detail. The best timing for me would be during June 2010.

CHAPTER 14

A Life Changing Experience

Ever since I have been diagnosed with cancer and throughout my treatment, I have had many conversations with all sorts of people, both close friends, family and many strangers. Oftentimes, comments have been made that having cancer must give me time to reflect on life and perhaps make some potentially life changing decisions. It has been making me think.

Before I became a teacher, which was only a few years ago, I had a successful career in marketing in the mobile phone industry. I had worked for Orange and 3, both through the launch of their networks, which was pretty hectic to say the least. After we had Marcus we had a 'live out' nanny, as I was earning considerably more than John at the time, it seemed silly for me not to carry on working. The fact that I had also discovered that babies didn't really interest me that much may also have been a major contributory factor!

Then my mother became very ill and died of metastatic cancer of the spine and lungs, which had spread from breast cancer. She had her lumpectomy on my thirty-ninth birthday – the same day I left Orange. I was working for 3 when she died and they were incredibly generous allowing me six weeks off work to spend with Mum and manage the arrangements afterwards. She died on the 1st April 2003. That will always make me laugh as it had been Mother's Day only two days before. Imagine if she had died on that day! I would never have been able to enjoy Mother's Day in the same way again. However, bless her, she held on till April Fool's Day, so now I can have a little chuckle to myself each year, knowing that she would have taken great amusement from dying on such an auspicious day.

This was a huge catalyst in my life and made me rethink all sorts of things, most especially my family and its importance. I had two lovely children and barely got to see them. Emma, our fantastic Nanny, was getting to spend more time with my children than I was. I worked very long hours and had to commute to Maidenhead each day. 3 had become a disaster company and the dream job I had been promised there turned out to be a nightmare, as the network launch was too early and my job became crisis management instead of customer relationship management. What was I doing? Why did I have children if I was never getting to spend any time with them? I was always so tired.

By June that year I knew I needed to make a change in my life and do something different, but what? I handed in my notice and left work at the end of August. Emma left us, which was a great wrench for the children, but she will always be part of our family (Marcus calls her number two mummy) and Lizzie and Marcus were bridesmaid and page boy at her wedding. I had to learn to be a full time mum. Marcus was five and Lizzie seven.

For a few months I did all sorts of different types of volunteer work at school, including being chair of the PTA. I became a parent reading partner with some of the older children, helped with the library, managed the sale of school uniform and undertook any project they could find me to do. I also became a volunteer at St Luke's Hospice. I worked in the Harrow shop one afternoon a week and did some PR work for the fundraising department one morning a week. I also discovered that although babies didn't interest me that much, I was now really enjoying my own children. Having the time with them, I actually got to know them so much better.

Financially it was quite hard that year and we had to increase the mortgage, but John was so supportive and I adore him for giving me the gift of a year not working, to help me make my mind up about what I wanted to do.

By Christmas I was pretty sure I wanted to retrain as a primary school teacher. I had, when I had done my degree, thought about teaching PE at secondary level, but had gone back to a marketing career instead, so John was not surprised. Others, however, were. I am not very patient and so many of the family thought I would never have the patience to teach, or that I would not want to be a class teacher for long, preferring instead to climb the management ladder. If I became a teacher it would also mean that I would get so much more time with the children, especially as I would be at their school. I would also get to see all their assemblies and performances without having to take any time off work!

So the head teacher encouraged me and I applied to train on the graduate teacher programme (GTP) at my children's school and successfully gained a place. This meant I worked for a year in school, with one afternoon a week release at the University of Hertfordshire and at the end of the year if I passed I would be a qualified teacher. This is what I did and I have been at the same school ever since. After my training year I worked part time four days a week and then in my second year I dropped down to two. I did this so that I had time for my other passion, which was St Luke's Hospice. As an organisation they were trying to make the board of trustees a much more organised and cohesive team. They did this by recruiting individuals with a broad range of skills which the hospice required to ensure it had proper governance. I applied at the end of my teacher training year and following a panel interview, succeeded in being appointed to one of the three vacancies.

So, as you can see, I had pretty much totally changed my life around already. How would having cancer myself make me change any more? Friends and family were right; I had become ambitious about moving up the management ladder, because I had all the management experience in business to translate to education. I also

I FELT A RIGHT ONE...

missed the challenge of greater responsibility, however, having read so many books and knowing from working one day a week as acting deputy head how pressurised a management job in school can be. I am starting to rethink how quickly I might want to do this.

Perhaps I should just stay a class teacher for a while. It is a job I love and actually making a difference on a day to day basis with children is so deeply satisfying that I am reluctant to give that up totally.

It is something to think about before the summer when I go back to work.

There have been some other noticeable changes for me, but more about that later.

CHAPTER 15

The End of the Poison and Time to Get Nuked!

It is now the end of March 2009 and I am due to have my last chemo on the 31st. I really don't want any more delays and had asked at the last one whether they would reduce the dose, as I had had two sessions in a row delayed. They felt, however, as it was my last one that there was no point.

I go for my blood tests and, amazingly, all is OK and I can receive my poison for the very last time. I have brought with me a thank you note, some hand cream and chocolates for Mary and Rommel and I say an emotional goodbye at the end. It is hard to explain the kind of relationship you develop with the medical staff who are treating you for cancer. I am sure it may be the same for patients with any other major life threatening diseases. However, as I only have experience of cancer, I can only comment on that. You build up a bond, because they are helping you through such a critical part of your life, whether you like it or not. The move to the next treatment changes how you feel about the cancer. Were there any cells left? Have they all been destroyed? Only time will tell.

I now have to wait a month before I can start radiotherapy. Over the next few weeks I have a variety of medical appointments. I go and see my GP again, as I now need to arrange to have my coil removed. Sorry if this is too much information for some you, but the reason is important. I had gone on the Mirena coil a few years ago, when I became menopausal, in order to reduce the heaviness of my periods and reduce the pain. This coil, however, contains progesterone and it is now time to get it removed. My cancer is progesterone receptive and we must make sure that I am not receiving any unecessary hormones which may encourage the growth of any errant cancer cells. Besides, one of the great, and I mean *great*, benefits of chemo is that if you are menopausal, it will most likely finish you off and you won't have any more periods. Yippee! So I need to have the coil taken out anyway, as I really don't need it now. This also has to happen before I can start taking the Tamoxifen.

The doctor tries, but cannot remove it. I see two other female GPs at the surgery over the next two weeks and they cannot remove it either. Each time is not a pleasant experience, as they are trying to pull something out that has become quite attached to the inside of your womb! They say I need to get my oncologist to refer me to a gynaecological specialist to have it removed and that I may need a scan to identify why and where it is stuck.

It is now the Easter holidays and the children and I go visiting a whole range of people, who have taken the time to come and see me over the last few months. Over Easter itself, Justin (my youngest brother) and Jo, Jono, Harry and Katie come to visit, which is great for Lizzie and Marcus. Normally we have quite a hectic social life, as I do live by the maxim, 'work hard, play hard'. This year has obviously been different though, because we didn't know how well or not I would feel at any one time, so we have done a lot less gallivanting around the country seeing friends and family than we would normally have done. I can see Lizzie and Marcus appreciating that the worst part of my treatment is coming to an end and that their social life is also improving.

During the holidays, the den at the bottom of the garden is

finished and the children and I visit Ikea to sort out some simple furnishing then move the drums down from the loft. I build most of the furniture and when John is around he moves the futon out of the loft so there is a sofa down there for the kids to chill out on.

The week we go back to school I have two appointments at Mount Vernon Cancer Centre, where I am to have my radiotherapy. The first visit is to the Linda Jackson Centre, which is a charity that supports patients through the treatment process by providing, psychological, emotional and physical support with alternative therapies. I go to a talk about the actual process of having radiotherapy, how it works and how it might make me feel. This is really useful and I now feel more prepared for what is to come next.

Some people say radio is worse than chemo. Maybe that is because you are so tired and low after the chemo that radio feels like you are adding insult to injury, or maybe it is because you actually have to go to hospital every day for treatment and for me that will be three weeks. This can be a bit of a chore. Apparently it is the tiredness which people feel is cumulative and also that your skin can get really sore.

The next day we have more visitors from France, someone I have known since I was sixteen and again getting to spend time with old friends is a wonderful tonic. After they have left, I have my planning visit with the radiographers who are going to prepare me for radiotherapy. I go to Mount Vernon where I have a CT scan, so that they can decide on the exact area that is going to receive the radiation. At this point they triangulate me, which is where they tattoo me with three blue dots, one under each arm and one in the middle of my chest. I had always wanted a tattoo, but never been brave enough to get one done, and now I had three all in one go. I had achieved a lifetime's ambition! Admittedly they were tiny, but they were still permanent. These three dots are essential so that every time I am given the radiation, it is in exactly the same place. I feel like a human theodolite or trig point! They ask me my preferred time for treatment and I say as early in the morning as possible

I FELT A RIGHT ONE…

would be best. At least this way I don't waste so much of the day and I get it over and done with as soon as possible. I am booked in to start on Tuesday 6th May at 9.00am.

I make the most of the next week and get lots organised and sorted, just in case the radio lays me low. I have actually been preparing for the Hatch End Triathlon. I have swum a few times now and have even managed a couple of runs, of only about a mile, but runs nevertheless. Annie Wheelie recommends ice baths for my feet after running. John had ice bathed his whole body whilst training for the London Marathon. I try this for my feet and sit at the PC and read stuff whilst my feet are in an ice bath of water on the floor. I hope the distraction of working/reading/playing on the PC will make the whole experience more tolerable. Not so.

On the Tuesday evening in the last week of April, I attend a recently set up group arranged by Elaine Sasto, the breast care nurse at the Clementine Churchill Hospital. The group is made up of women who have all had either a single or double mastectomy. Most have gone through chemo and radio and some are still in the process of treatment. Some women have had the disease more than once.

We are a little squashed in the small physio room, but it is great to talk to so many different women who have all had a similar experience to me. We are asking each other questions, sharing experiences, sharing the niggling side effects of treatment that drive us mad but which other people would think we were daft to complain about. The meetings are going to be organised for about every six weeks or so and Elaine is going to arrange different visitors that relate to what we have all been through. At this first meeting someone from Clarins comes along to talk about the type of make-up you can use to help combat the hair loss (eyebrows and eyelashes) and other effects on your skin from chemo. I am surprised at how much I find I enjoyed the evening. I feel that I have so much support from my friends that I don't need the support from strangers. However, the mutual experience, I also got the impression from the others, was beneficial for all of us.

The End of the Poison and Time to Get Nuked!

That week, following the third visit to my GP to get my coil extracted, I arrange with my oncologist a referral to a gynaecologist, to investigate the best way to get my coil removed. I have an appointment at the end of this week, before I start radiotherapy next week. I also catch up with an old uni friend I have not seen for 20 years and an old school friend. My social life is still continuing on the up and up.

On Friday, I see an excellent female gynaecologist. My oncologists' secretary had asked if I preferred a male or female doctor. I had opted for female, as I was starting to get a bit tired of showing the most intimate parts of my body off to male doctors. I felt I deserved a change and asked for a referral to a lady. Miss Pitkin is great and very down to earth. She has one go, and out pops the coil. No need for any more complex procedures. She also arranges for me to have a blood test so my hormone levels can be checked before I start taking any long term drugs. This will help assess whether I have truly finished going through the menopause. I leave the hospital happy that I am ready for my next stage of treatment.

At about this time, four weeks since I completed my chemotherapy, a wonderful thing is starting to happen: my hair is starting to grow back. It is really soft, fuzzy hair, but hair nevertheless. It is a wonderful feeling to know that my body is starting to heal itself after receiving so much poison. John and the children love feeling the downy fur and for the first time in my life I don't mind people playing with my hair. It is also about this time, I have someone actually comment to me about it.

I am filling my car with petrol one day and am paying in the shop, when the attendant smiles at me and says, "A nice hair cut for the summer?"

Without thinking I reply. "No. Cancer and chemotherapy," I know I shouldn't have been so blunt, but I just didn't expect the question. The poor man is so embarrassed, but I try to put him at ease when he apologises and tell him he was not to know, that actually it is growing back now so that is good. He politely asks if I am OK now and I am able to put his mind at rest with an enthusiastic, "Absolutely brilliant, thank you!"

At the weekend, we go down to the West Country, as John and the kids are going to run in the Glastonbury Fun Run, along with several friends. John is running the 10K, Lizzie 5K and Marcus 3K. All have a good but tiring time and then it's back to the house for a barbecue. It is the first May bank holiday the next day, so we stay over again and leisurely make our way back to London the next day.

Tuesday morning arrives and I get myself up to Mount Vernon Hospital Cancer Centre for my 9.00am radiotherapy session. I check in and am sent round to wait in one of the small waiting rooms that they have outside each of the radiotherapy rooms. As this is my first session the staff explain absolutely everything that is happening, as it happens. As the previous patient is getting themselves sorted out at the end of their treatment, you are ushered to stand outside the huge door. This is when you realise how strong the radiation must actually be. The door is about 30cm thick and is shut whilst each patient is irradiated. When the previous patient walks out, you walk in. You have to take your clothes off the top half of your body and then lie down on the table underneath the scanner. As you have to remain totally still and in the same position for each treatment, they use the three blue, tattooed dots to get you into the correct position. To ensure that they do not irradiate any part of your body that should not receive it, they put your arms into arms rests, above and to either side of your head. This is actually the worst part, as my right arm finds it hard to get into this position without causing pain in my chest. The scar tissue where my breast used to be is so tight, that when I put my arms too far back it stretches the skin so it actually hurts. However, it is only for a few short minutes so should not be too bad.

I ask one of the radiographers, of which there are two, how strong the radiation is. He comments that it is ten times as strong as a normal x-ray, but stays on for several minutes, whereas a normal x-ray, take less than a second. So, by my reckoning, for four minutes of radiotherapy you are receiving approximately 2,400 times as much radioactivity than you would with a run of the mill x-ray. I am going to have this done fifteen times, which is roughly the equivalent of 36,000 x-rays. Mmmm, that's a lot of radiation. No wonder the door is so thick if you are working with this all the time, then you would certainly need the protection. It is reassuring that there are two radiographers and I hear them discussing all the measurements of where they need to locate the radiation and double checking them. I am glad they take these safety measures, as when you are playing around with such large doses of potentially dangerous treatment, you certainly don't want to get it wrong.

As soon as I am ready the medical staff leave the room and the very large door starts to shut. When it is completely closed a voice comes over the intercom to tell me to be as still as possible. They irradiate me twice, once from the side and once from overhead. The scanner moves automatically between each bout. All in all, it takes less than five minutes.

Whilst I am getting dressed, one of the radiographers gives me a tube of special aqueous cream to rub onto the area of my chest that is being irradiated, twice a day. This should help reduce the likelihood of my skin getting sore. Before I leave this first session, a nurse comes to see me to ask if I would be interested in taking part in some research about cancer. I agree to participate and we go to a room where she takes some blood and some basic details and gives me the questionnaire which I will need to complete and return in a postage paid envelope. She explains that it is anonymous, but to be honest, I don't actually care. If I could do anything that would shed light on the causes of cancer so that someone else would not have to go through what I am, then as far as I am concerned they could post my name in 20m high letters on the side of the hospital. I take the questionnaire home to peruse. One radiotherapy down and fourteen to go.

That evening I send out an email inviting everyone to a party on the 4th July to celebrate the end of my treatment. This is something

I FELT A RIGHT ONE...

that I have been thinking about for a while and I really want to do. Planning it and inviting everyone makes me really feel like the treatment is coming to an end and that is something to celebrate, surely. Mind you, I don't need much persuasion as I would celebrate anything with anyone, anytime.

Each morning that week I go for my treatment and am done by 10.00am most days. I am in school on the Thursday and have a meeting at St Luke's that week as well, so I'm just keeping myself ticking over. By Friday my skin is starting to get a little red but I am not feeling too bad, so I decide to go ahead with my participation in the Hatch End Triathlon.

CHAPTER 16

A Girl's Got to Do What a Girl's Got to Do

Some more background here. The Hatch End Triathlon is not really a full triathlon; it falls into the sprint category and is, in fact, really a super sprint. The swim is 400m, the cycle is 17km and the run is a pleasingly short 3k. The first time I did it in was May 2006 when I was 44. I came 151st out of 151 adult athletes in just over an hour and a half. In other words, I came last. The following year, 2007, I again came 151st but was not last, as this time there were 163 entries, with a slightly faster time of 1 hour, 29 minutes and 9 seconds. In 2008 I didn't participate as I had a shoulder injury, but this year no mere chemotherapy and radiotherapy are going to stop me. It is just something I have to do. Not for anyone else, but just for me. I just have to prove to myself that I have the mental strength to complete it. I know it won't be fast or pretty, but it has to be done.

A whole bunch of friends and my children are also competing. We have to be up horribly early, as you have to register an hour before your start time and I am due in the pool at about 7.30am. This is the first year that they are using electronic timing and as we enter the pool you collect you ankle bracelet to wear for the duration of the race. In order to be able to run in this event comfortably, I have always had to wear a sports bra under my swimsuit, so that I don't hurt myself. This means that wearing the bra to hold my swim prosthesis does not feel any different than before. I strip off down to my bra and swimsuit and then walk in bare feet to the swimming pool to wait my turn. I have to leave my glasses with someone at the exit end of the pool and wait in line to start my swim.

Even though I have no hair, I still have to wear a swim hat in the pool, so that the lap counters can use your individually coloured headpiece to identify how many times you have swum up and down. Hatch End Pool is an old twenty-five yard pool (indeed it is the very pool I learnt to swim in) and so you have to swim seventeen lengths to complete 400m. Normally I would swim only front crawl, but I find myself swimming a couple of lengths of backstroke just to catch my breath. Also, when there are about eight of you in one lane you have to overtake and let people overtake you if necessary. They do try to organise you into swim groups of about the same ability speed wise, but when people complete their entry forms, I am not really sure how accurately they know their swim speed. Obviously the elite and normally competitive triathletes do, but the nature of this event attracts a lot of people like me who do not normally complete triathlons, so their time estimates may not be as accurate. I swim fairly well to time and don't get overtaken. In fact, I have to overtake a couple of people, so I am really pleased.

I collect my glasses and gently jog out of the pool back to transition to collect my bike. I swiftly don a t-shirt, leggings and put my cycle helmet on and walk/jog my bike out to the Uxbridge Road. I get on my bike and start peddling as fast as I can, which is not really too fast. The cycle is my worst part normally; I don't really have a particularly fast bike and this year I have done almost no training whatsoever. It is three laps of the roughly triangular route. Whilst cycling up George V Avenue, Johnnie Wheelie is sitting in the grassy central reservation of the dual carriageway on a deck chair with a saucepan and wooden spoon, banging and shouting for all he is worth. It is a great boost to the moral and makes me smile knowing I will get to see him a couple more times. He is staying near home to watch as he is preparing stuff for Anne's fiftieth birthday party this afternoon.

Twice more round the route then I finally get off my bike and jog, well by now I am actually walking it, back to transition. I remove my helmet and jog out onto the grass for the final killer leg: the run. This time it really is the killer. I end up walking about half of the time because I am so shattered. I can hardly breathe and I really wonder what on earth I am doing, but I have to finish. I can hear the kids, Sarah and several other people shouting my name in encouragement and it really does work. Each time they shout I find myself trying to jog, rather than walk. Ed (Sarah's husband) has already finished and is cheering me on right at the end. The last few hundred metres I run as fast as my very tired legs will carry me and lunge over the finish line. I am spent, my throat is closing up and I feel like I can't breathe. Ed walks over and gives me a huge hug and congratulates me and a few tears spill down my face. I have done it. I have finished it and despite feeling physically drained, I am elated that I have managed to complete the race. Yes, I would have liked to have actually run the whole run, but who am I trying to kid, the run is always the hardest and with so little training and being so physically depleted at the moment, what was I expecting?

John is still out racing, as are the other friends. I wrap myself up and stand to cheer them on. When all the adults have finished, there is a short changeover time where all the adults have to clear everything out of transition and then the children put all their equipment in and get ready. It is lunchtime by the time the children have finished. They are both pleased with their performance. Before we leave, we are able to check our times. I completed the course in 1 hour 42 minutes and 41 seconds and came 209th out of 213 adults. I have not come last and even though about nearly fourteen minutes slower than last time, I am incredibly happy with what I have achieved. I know I will be able to complete the nine mile midnight walk for St Luke's in a month's time without any problem. Time to start collecting the pledges.

I FELT A RIGHT ONE...

We go home and I relax in a warm bath and then get dressed up to go to the the Wheelies for Anne's birthday party. It is a really fun afternoon catching up with lots of very old friends and people I haven't seen for a while. All of us that had competed in the morning are a little tired and careworn, but we blag seats whenever we can and a few drinks helps us relax.

Again I do wonder why I needed to do this. Certainly those that care about me had also been asking me the same thing? For me it is so important to have goals to focus on and this triathlon was a goal which was unrelated to my health. Focusing on something physical which is not related to the cancer has allowed me to do something healthy that makes your body hurt and ache, rather than just having treatments that do the same thing. Psychologically, it is a huge boost as well. To know that even under such pressure my body has been able to cope helps me realise that I will heal quickly and recover from the negative effects of both chemo and radio. Really I just needed to prove to myself that I had the mental strength to cope. If I can do this, I can do anything.

CHAPTER 17

The Treatment Comes to an End

On Monday begins my second week of radiotherapy, and it is fairly uneventful. I have started getting to know a few of the people who have their sessions at about the same time as me. One in particular, a young Czech girl who is only twenty-five. Again I think myself lucky, as I cannot imagine going through this at such a young age. She is really positive and we get on really well. She lives up in Luton though, so it would not be easy for us to get together. Working and studying, is proving it quite tough, nevertheless, she has a really positive outlook and her hair, like mine, is just starting to grow back again. It is definitely helpful to have someone that you look forward to seeing when going for your treatment, it makes it seem more social and less medical.

I catch up with three different friends, including Xenia, my colleague from school, then at the weekend it is my Father-in-Law's Seventieth Birthday. It is all round to my in-laws for a family barbecue. I also complete and return the questionnaire that I was given last week. I actually have to undertake some research about what my grandparents died of. I know how my maternal grandmother had died as I was eighteen, but Mum's dad had died when I was only about seven and both my father's parents had died before I was born. As it turns out, my paternal grandmother had died of ovarian cancer at only fifty-six and I had never known. Chris,

I FELT A RIGHT ONE...

my eldest brother, knew all of this and was able to fill in all the gaps in my knowledge. I can only hope that the information helps in some way.

This week I also start to take the drug Tamoxifen. I couldn't take it any earlier as I needed to wait until the coil had been removed, then of course I had started radiotherapy and David Fermont wanted to make sure that I didn't suffer any ill effects from that first. If I had started the two treatments at the same time, he would not know which one was causing a problem if I had actually had one. So I start to take the drug and know that this is something I am going to be doing every day for the next five years; if not this drug then one that has a similar effect.

As I am going to be taking this drug for up to five years, I think it is a good idea to read the leaflet inside the box which explains the side effects in some detail. I had looked at this before last year when I took it for a month before my surgery, but now I really consider it properly. I know that one of the side effects is possible deep vein thrombosis (DVT), which is why I will have to take aspirin the day before I go on any long haul flight, as well as wearing those sexy compression stockings, to counteract this potential effect. The list is a lot longer than this however: hot flushes, breast pain or discomfort (especially at the start of treatment), skin rash, dry skin, hair loss or thinning, itching in the genital area, stomach upsets, weight gain, swelling due to water retention, dizziness, tiredness, confusion, depression and headaches. It can also affect periods, which won't bother me as I doubt I will have any after chemo anyway. The piéce de resistance is a slightly increased risk of cancer of the womb in women who take it for a long time. There were some other nasty potential effects and I have also been told, joint pain, particularly in the lower body. What a lovely bunch! The irony that the drug helping to reduce the risk of of the breast cancer recurring might give you uterine cancer has to make you laugh. Only time will tell, what effects, if any, Tamoxifen is going to have on me.

The Treatment Comes to an End

Next week, I am quite busy, I attend a meeting at the Institute of Education and commit myself to completing an assignment based on some training I had last year, which will start me on the road to a masters degree. I work a day in school, attend Lizzie's parents' evening and have coffee with friends. On Saturday morning we drop the children off at John's sister's (Ann) then drive down to Llandovery for a charity ball. We have to be up early in the morning to drive back to London for a family first communion and party. It is the second bank holiday weekend in May and the beginning of half term, so we stay late into the evening as there is no rush to get the children home to bed.

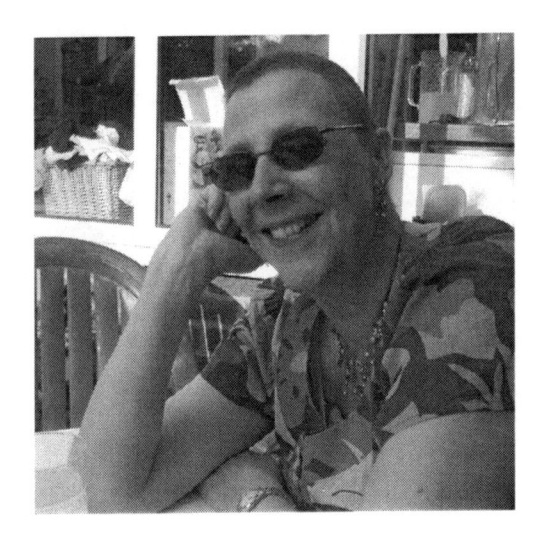

Baby hair! Eight weeks post chemo

We have a restful bank holiday and I now only have two more days of radiotherapy. I am glad, because the skin on my chest is beginning to get a little sore and I am now feeling more than a little tired. Not as bad as I had expected though, which is good. I have not swam since the triathlon in case the chlorine irritated my skin and it is a shame, because even with the exercises I feel the skin on my chest getting tighter. This makes it more painful each time I have radiotherapy, when I have to stretch my arms back and put them in the arm rests. Thank goodness I only have two sessions left.

I FELT A RIGHT ONE...

Each year for the last five or six years John and I have gone away overnight with Jane and Tony to play two rounds of golf. I am a little worried about playing for the first time after having my mastectomy. How will the tightness of the skin across my chest affect my swing? Will I be able to make a full swing? Normally we play boys versus girls, as I am a handicap to whoever I play with, which means I need to play with the best player, Jane.

For the first time since we started this tradition, the girls win. Amazingly, my swing is much more consistent. I think it is because I am worried about my chest I don't try to overhit the ball. I am precise, straight and most importantly I score thirty-four stableford points!

CHAPTER 18

Getting Back to Normal and the Waiting Game

So, now all of my treatment, apart from taking drugs, is complete. Any more that I have done will be my own choice for reconstruction, or if I get a recurrence of cancer. I am confident it is going to be the former and not the latter. It will be six months, the end of the year, before I can think about reconstruction, so it is time to get my life back to normal whilst I wait. I am still catching up with friends, knowing that I go back to work on the 6th July for the last two weeks of term. I do start to ramp up work a little bit and go back in to teach my class PSHE (personal, social and health education), in particular sex education, once a week. This is my favourite subject and it is great to be back in the classroom spending time with the children.

I continue to attend the breast care group and we have some interesting visitors, including the owner of Rigby and Pellor (the lingerie company), where I have been buying my bras for the last twenty years. She is a remarkable lady, who does not look her age and who is happy to lift her top up and show us her reconstruction following breast cancer. We have a reconstructive surgeon come and talk to us and a stylist to talk about how we dress – so covering a really broad range of topics.

I FELT A RIGHT ONE...

In June I take part in the St Luke's Hospice Midnight Walk. For a variety of reasons I end up doing it on my own. My mother-in-law and some of her friends are there, but I want to walk it as fast as I can and get home to bed! Having got everyone to sponsor me for shaving my head only a few months ago, I do not in all conscience feel I can go and ask everyone again. However, I do try and in the end gain £140 of sponsorship; I even get my oncologist David Fermont to chip in.

It is an amazing evening. The Byron Hall at the back of the Harrow Leisure Centre is taken over by over 1,000 pink-clad women. I find reading the messages written about why people are walking very moving. A large number are walking for women who died from breast cancer, something that could have happened to me, but didn't. We set off at midnight and once the rush along the narrow pavements at the start has finished, the line of pink ladies spreads out over a very long distance. It is nine miles from start to finish and goes through Stanmore, Queensbury and back through Kenton past the Hospice itself. I have brought an iPod so I plug myself firmly in and walk as fast as I possibly can. I manage it in 2 hours and 10 minutes and am amongst some of the first people back to the leisure centre.

The whole way round we are supported and marshalled by a whole range of people, including some kind and enthusiastic young Asian lads who have come from one of the temples that supports St Luke's. They are fantastic and everytime you walk past one of them, they say something encouraging and give you a smile. I find the whole experience extremely uplifting and motivating.

By the time I finish I am really tired, but still buzzing as I drive home to a dark, unlit house and creep into bed. Fortunately, my physical tiredness overcomes my post walk high to allow me to go to sleep.

At the end of June we arrange to go to Edinburgh for the weekend to catch up with friends, whom we have not seen since they moved back to Scotland about ten years ago. A colleague of

Getting Back to Normal and the Waiting Game

mine, Linda, is going to come and stay for the weekend to look after the children. She had been offering for ages as she wants to do something to say thank you for having her to stay for several weeks when she first arrived in the UK from New Zealand. We decide to take her up on it.

We leave for Luton on Friday evening, but our flight is delayed by a couple of hours. By the time we get to Edinburgh Airport it is nearly 10.00pm. I recognise Marie and Jo as soon as I see them and they have not changed a bit.

We have a fantastic weekend. Being shown around by natives is definitely the best way to see a city. It is so relaxing being with such dear friends and we walk round the city, drive to the coast and generally eat and drink ourselves silly. I notice now, as my hair is starting to grow back, that people don't stare at me as much. I just look like I have a purposefully short hairstyle.

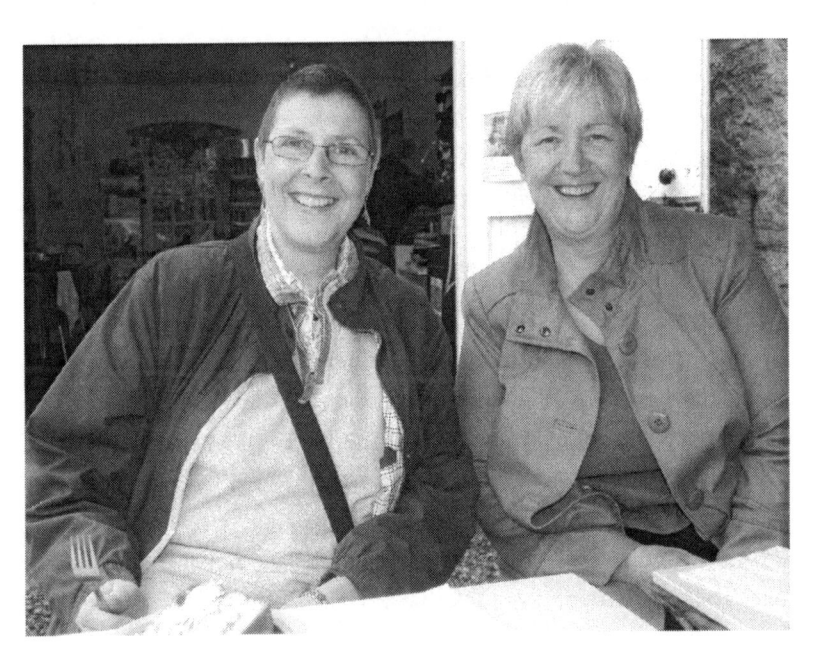

Me and Marie having some cake! Twelve weeks post chemo hair.

I FELT A RIGHT ONE...

Early in July we have the party to celebrate the end of all my treatment and use it as an opportunity to say thank you to everyone for all their support. I had sent out the invitations in early May and we were now expecting well over 100 people.

I have planned the food, John is going to cook a vegetarian curry and I am going to cook a chilli, then Waitrose will supply the rest. We use up a load of our Tesco vouchers to buy some champagne and other wine. We are really lucky with the weather; we borrow a couple of tables and some chairs and put up two pop-up gazebos. Friends come from far and wide and the party goes very well, apart from the fact that I have slightly over-catered, well that may be an understatement. I find myself giving food away to friends and neighbours as they leave, taking some into school on the Monday as well.

By the end of the evening I am shattered, but very happy. I find, when everyone has gone, that people have left me presents. I am so surprised and grateful, but I kind of wish they hadn't done and feel a little guilty, as it was not that kind of party. But if people want to give you presents, then you need to let them.

On the following Monday I go back to work full time, though not in class, as the children have got someone with them till the end of term. It is so good to be back at work. I realise how much I have missed being part of something. I know I have not been away the whole time, but as I have said before you miss so much of the day to day minutiae which makes the school tick if you only work part time. I am glad that I am not in class, as I think I would find that a bit tiring, but working my way back in like this is a great way to start. These two weeks also give me the chance to get everything sorted with my management role, ready for the beginning of next year. This is also the end of my time as acting deputy head, so I also make sure that I pass over any jobs that I have been doing that I will not have the time to do in the next academic year.

The week following the party John starts a new job. He had really discovered through my illness and treatment that travelling

Getting Back to Normal and the Waiting Game

so much and not being around had proven very tough for him and so he was leaving Rexam and moving to working in Slough for ICI. A much shorter journey when in the UK and little or no travelling.

In early July, Sarah has to have some surgery and she is sent to the same hospital that I was in. When I go to visit her, which nurse should be in her room? Cleo! It is really great to see her and for her to see me well. She gives me a big hug and has a short chat with me and Sarah as well. Cleo has seen me bald during chemo and she comments on how nicely my hair is growing back.

I now start my regimen of check-ups, which will be every three months. This will alternate between Michael Burke and David Fermont. I will have to have a mammogram once a year and perhaps an MRI every two to three years. These check-ups will go on for at least five years. Each time you go to see the doctor it makes you think about what they might find. I know in my heart of hearts that I am fine and that the visits are just a formality really, but what your heart knows and your head thinks can sometimes be completely different.

The way I deal with the visits is twofold. In terms of questions, I have my book in which I note down anything I want to ask. This means I don't have to remember them and also means I tend to forget about the visits until they actually come around. The second thing I do is try to treat them a bit like a social catch up. I know that sounds bizarre, but I feel I have developed a good relationship with both of my doctors. The fact that I am fairly brazen and ask lots of question about whether they have children or not, hobbies etc, means that I continue these conversations with them during each visit. Poor chaps, I must drive them completely mad, but it keeps my mind off why I am really going to see them.

It is then the summer holidays and we are going to Spain with Eammon, Zoe and the family. On our return from Spain, we discover that my brother Justin and family have been unable to have their summer holiday, as my sister-in-law's mother is really poorly and is not expected to live much longer. We offer to have the children for a while. It is great fun having them to stay and we try to keep them as busy as possible.

In no time it is early September and time to go back to school. There are two days training and then the children come back on Monday 7th September. This year I am working in year six for the first time. As term gets into full swing I start another module of my master's degree. This requires me to attend a lecture at the Harrow Teachers Centre every three weeks or so, to do homework and then next summer I will have to write a 10,000 word assignment. I like keeping busy and this is certainly going to help me achieve that.

John has now settled into his new job and is enjoying not travelling all the time, but because of the change our medical insurance cover also alters. I know that all the treatment I have had, I would have also had on the NHS, but the doctors I have been seeing have both retired from the NHS and I would like to keep seeing them. As it turns out, slightly ironically, David Fermont retires that December and Michael Burke follows him in March 2010, so all the efforts of sorting out the insurance didn't help me keep the two doctors I wanted to see. Who can blame them? They have both worked long and hard. Good doctors, like in any profession, go that extra mile and both of mine were well considered by most people that I knew, including friends and colleagues at St Luke's. I wish them both the very best for a long, happy and fulfilling retirement. Maybe I am just jealous and wish that I could retire now as well!

I am at the time of life where I am regularly attending fiftieth birthday parties and they are now coming thick and fast. We always joke that John is the baby in our friendship groups. This is because I cradle snatched! John is five and a half years younger than I am. They say you are only as old as the man you feel, so that makes me forty-two rather than nearly forty-eight!

I like to shock people when I tell them how I met John. You see I have known him and Eammon since they were 15! I was going out with their PE teacher at the time; I used to go and watch their rugby matches with the teacher. After leaving school, John and Eammon joined the rugby club that I socialised at and so when John was twenty-four and I was thirty, we actually started dating. We have been together ever since!

When half term comes round, we have a holiday to Scotland and then we start to re-invigorate our social life with gusto. Although you may find it hard to believe from what I have written, it really had actually taken a little bit of a dive during all my treatment. Ray (John's ex boss) and Angela come down from Yorkshire with Steve and Ann, some friends of theirs. Along with the Wheelies we go to see England v Argentina at Twickenham. The rugby is desperately poor and the most exciting part of the match is when the commentator asks the crowd not to throw paper airplanes made from the advertising card placed on every seat in the stadium, to see how far onto the pitch they can get them. We go up to London for some dinner and have an excellent evening at Belgos in Covent Garden. I really get to spend time with both Ray and Angela on this visit, something I have not had the pleasure of doing before.

I get the chance to say thank you to Ray. I had written to him the year before, just after I had my mastectomy, but I wanted to say it to him in person. It is impossible to say how much his support had helped John and I. He gave John as much time as he needed for me. He was flexible and totally understanding when John needed to change things, to go to appointments with me, or work from home. Ray is the kind of manager that everyone would like to have – a truly caring person who understands that although work is important, it is not the be all and end all of everything. I want to thank him for not making John worry, any more than any conscientious person would, about missing work or having to let other members of the team take the strain. Knowing that John was working for Ray and how supportive he was being eased my guilt. OK I hear you thinking, *why are you feeling guilty about having cancer?* But it is true. You do feel guilty about the huge upheaval, both emotionally and practically, it has on everyone around you. If you didn't have the disease, they would not have to change their plans or be inconvenienced in any way. When you are dealing with all the fall out of the diagnosis and the treatment, I find it is something that I did feel. Being able to express face to face with Ray how grateful I am is quite emotional. I get teary, just thinking about how supportive he was.

The process of writing this book also has a similar effect. When I actually think about what people have done for me over the last couple of years, I am awestruck at how many friends, family, colleagues have given their time, energy, love and emotion. When I think of specific incidences of kindness that made, and are still making, a material difference to how either John or I have coped, I find it evokes an incredibly strong emotional response.

CHAPTER 19

A Smashing Time!

Whilst life is returning to normal, I do think back to what Michael Burke said about how quickly people forget what you have been through. I honestly find this a real benefit. In the eyes of most people, I have gotten over the worst part of having cancer and actually they are right. Yes, you have to have check-ups and that does remind you of the risks that are still a real possibility going forward, but truly the mastectomy, chemo and radio have to be the worst parts. Only if it comes back do I have to rethink this view. Life is returning to normal and yes I do plan to put myself through some major surgery next year, but that is then and this is now. Live for the present.

As normality resumes, you start to recognise what normal now feels like for you personally. You realise that some things, apart from the physical differences, have also changed. As I mentioned before, you get asked by lots of people if having cancer and recovering from it makes you want to change anything in your life. For me, I have already made such a huge change by leaving commerce that I don't really feel the need to reinvent myself again. However, I am starting to notice that some things in me have changed.

I have always had a temper, a short fuse in fact. This is definitely a family trait that I have worked hard at trying to minimise over the years, although I am sure John and the children would tell you differently. Now, you would think that having had a life threatening illness would make a person feel that life is too short to lose your temper and so become more mellow. For me it has had exactly the opposite effect. Instead of 'light blue touch paper and stand back', it is now, 'press the digital button for immediate explosion'.

I think my children have always found me a little schizophrenic, in that I will blow up over something and then thirty seconds later I am completely normal. I don't sulk, in fact I cannot bear it. I have always been like that, as my father was a world champion sulker and I swore I would never do that with anyone.

In early December 2009, John is about to go to the US for a few days for work. He is sitting in the lounge having a cup of coffee and reading the paper. He is also trying to swap over his SIM card from one phone to another without success. I don't realise this at the time. John is a creature of habit and his favourite thing to do on a Saturday morning is to sit down with a cup of freshly made coffee, made in his pride and joy of a coffee machine, and read *The Times*. This time is sacrosanct to him and he will not do anything during this half hour, weekly ritual. Normally he will sit at the kitchen table, but sometimes if there is some good sport on the TV he will park himself on the sofa and multitask for the only time in his life, by watching and reading about sport at the same time.

I go to the loo. We have a downstairs shower and utility room off the kitchen. I flush the loo with difficulty, as it has not really been working properly since about June or July and now there are at least two different things wrong with it. You have to realise that John's dad is a heating engineer and plumber, so getting a toilet sorted out should not be a difficult thing to do in our family. I have asked him innumerable times to ask his dad to sort it out. It has been so bad that we have had to leave the top of the cistern off and have a small hammer at the ready, to gently tap a part of the mechanism to make it stop overfilling itself when the cistern is full.

Now it is running like Niagra falls. It has had this extra problem for about three weeks, as I discovered when I was about to leave the house for school one day recently. I am a bit of an environmentally friendly nut, in fact John calls me the recycling Nazi, so as you can imagine leaving the house with a toilet that is flowing like a river is not something I can easily allow myself to do. I called John, who was on his way to work and who basically said 'what can he do' from there and that he would sort it out when he got home. I asked him if he would call his dad to ask him to come and mend it. He said he would, but then he has been saying that for about six months now!

So for the last three weeks the toilet has had to be tapped, banged and flushed multiple times before it will stop continually running with water. This Saturday morning it seems to be even worse. I call to John and ask if he will come and have a look.

"In a minute," is his terse reply.

I flush the toilet again at least three times, which takes a few minutes. I then walk into the lounge to see John reading the paper and drinking his coffee. I ask nicely again, "Will you please come and look at this toilet for me?"

"I said in a minute OK, I'm busy".

Yeah right, I think to myself, *busy reading the bloody paper, when I am stressing about this stupid toilet.* I go back and try again, to no avail. Three, four, five more flushes. I feel myself start to mentally fray around the edges. "John, could you please come and look at this stupid toilet for me?" I shout angrily.

"I told you I am busy and I will come in a minute", he shouts back, equally cross.

The fraying is complete and I totally lose it. "That's it!" I scream, "I have had it with this f***ing toilet, I am going to smash it to smithereens!"

I turn through the door of the shower room to the chest of drawers in the utility room which contain all our tools, systematically going through each draw before I find the small lump hammer used for minor demolition jobs around the house and garden.

I extricate the hammer, return to the shower room and just as my arm is plunging in its downward arc toward the cistern, John grabs my arm and shouts at the top of his voice, "What the hell do you think you are doing? Don't be so bloody ridiculous".

"I told you I am fed up with this toilet. What on earth do I have to do to get you to look at it?" I shout back.

A full scale argument ensues and I storm up to our bedroom in tears. We end up having a long discussion about John feeling like I am bullying him into doing something he doesn't want to do at that moment in time, whilst I express my dissatisfaction at the fact that he hasn't realised that I have no fuse anymore and that he needs to understand and make adjustments. I also tell him how unreasonable it is to have waited so long to get it sorted. He tells me I should have called his dad myself, or got a plumber in. My rationale is that I wouldn't have known how to explain to his father what was actually wrong with the loo and that anyway, if I had called another plumber in, his father would have been really cross.

This incident, although horrible at the time as I really don't like arguing with John, is what makes me realise that my ability to control my temper is much worse than it used to be. Not a positive change, it has to be said, not something I am proud of either. I try to analyse why this is the case and as I tell people the story of the toilet, it helps me to process the way my mind is now working. Most people find the story very funny and I am pleased to say, on the whole, I think I was very patient, for the six months previous to that fateful Saturday morning. John and I can also now look back and laugh at it.

It was a real catalyst for an important discussion that we should possibly have had earlier, but until something happens that actually makes you realise how you feel and you can, in a demonstrable way, show the people closest to you what psychological effects having cancer has actually manifested, it doesn't really register. Is it an excuse? I don't think so. I really feel that sometimes, definitely not all the time, life really is too short to put up with some of the crap that you are supposed to take in your stride. My stride is now more like a walk on uneven cobble stones which requires a skip now and then, rather than a steady pace.

I think that my patience is thinnest with the people closest to me. Is that because I expect them to understand me better and therefore make appropriate adjustments? I don't know. Perhaps it is because I know I am safe with them and that they will love me, no matter what I do. Of course I am still patient with the children at school, but inefficient customer service, especially with call centres, now seems to drive me even madder than it did before. Inanimate objects also raise my blood pressure much higher than I would like: PCs, photocopiers, dishwashers etc. often get shouted at as my frustration causes a miniature volcanic eruption, or reduces me to tears and sometimes, both. I do feel guilty that my family have to take the brunt of it, and I do try to control it but sometimes when the red mist comes down, I just have to give it its head and it burns out much quicker.

The other major change that I have noticed in myself which others may not have, is that I want to experience as much as I can in my life. Holidays, which have always been important, have become even more so. I want to travel and see so much. I want to spend time with my children before they grow up too much and give them some brilliant memories of their childhood. Material things have become less important; I find myself giving more presents of theatre and show tickets and the like. I find myself going to the theatre and concerts more myself, creating a shared history with my family that will always be there no matter what happens in the future.

CHAPTER 20

Planning

As the year comes to an end, it is time to start planning what I am going to do with regard to my reconstructive surgery. It makes me think again about what my motivation is for doing this. I do feel slightly selfish and a little self indulgent about what is in effect cosmetic surgery. However, it is more than that; it is not just myself I am putting through this, it will have an effect on lots of different people including my class, who I will have to leave for several weeks; my colleagues, who will have to pick up some of my work; my friends, whose support I will need, but last, and most importantly, John and the children. It will have a significant effect on them. They will have to put up with me being very immobile, needing support and not really having a proper summer holiday as I may not be capable of doing too much.

How do you make a decision as to whether you do or don't have something like this done? It is really major surgery, much more significant than the original mastectomy. The recovery time will be much longer and it feels selfish. Everyone tells me it isn't, but I cannot shake the feeling that I could manage without. The key word is 'manage'. Why should I just manage? Why shouldn't I try to get my body back to some level of normality? It doesn't bother me when I look in the mirror, it certainly doesn't seem to have affected how John feels about me physically and my children don't bat an eyelid when I walk round the house naked. Well not round the whole house, more like from bedroom to bathroom. They just don't like it when I leave my prosthesis on the stairs!

I have gone through an incredibly hot, horrible summer with sweat collecting behind the prosthesis and the hot flushes don't help. If I have the reconstruction then I can put all this behind me and have an almost normal figure again. In fact, although I will have big scars, once they have faded, my figure might even be improved.

One of the basic drivers is that I had felt, almost immediately after having the mastectomy, that I would want reconstruction. So it must be something that I feel at a subliminal level, almost an instinct that it is the right thing to do. I do understand that this may not be the right route for all women in my position, but for me I just feel it is something that I should do. Having said this, during the nineteen months between mastectomy and reconstructive surgery, my thoughts and feelings about whether or not I should get a new breast, continually vacillate. I just keep asking myself if it is really necessary. Yes of course it is. Should I really have it done? Why the hell not! What will I be letting myself in for? Ultimately getting a more normal body. So, John and I agree that I should 'go for it' and I start to make plans.

One of the problems with having private medical cover is when it stops. John had changed jobs in the summer and had gone from manufacturing aluminium cans to making paint instead and we have to wait for the medical cover to kick in. When he changed jobs he had to make sure that the new insurer would accept me as a member of the scheme, knowing how expensive I was going to be to them. To their credit they did accept me, but it means I have to go through all sorts of discussions and case histories again and learn all the new processes of the different company.

The reason I care so much about staying private is that it would allow me to control the time when I have the surgery and give me continuity of medical care, including the original surgeon, my oncologist (both of whose care I would be in for the next five years) and also the plastic surgeon. Having developed a relationship with all these medics it is not something that I wanted to go through all over again.

Being a teacher and working in a year six class, means I do have some moral responsibility to the children. It is a very important year for them, not just because of the nationals SATs tests but because it is their last year in primary school, so it is really important to prepare them for secondary school. Also, because I have the class who I started with last year, they had been so disrupted with three other teachers taking them when I went off sick that I want to mess them around as little as possible. I want to time the surgery to when it will have the least impact on the children. To me that would be at the end of the summer term, after they have done all their tests and I have taught the most important parts of the curriculum. It will also mean that I will have to have less time off school which has to be better for the school and also for me.

So in December 2009, I write to Adam Searle again to say I am ready to start planning the reconstruction process and get him to complete the required paperwork for the insurance company. Christmas comes and goes, with the excitement of a reunion of four girls who were at university together, from Canada, the Midlands and Streatham! We have a fantastic time and our poor partners are probably bored silly by the discussions, but they don't show it and we have a fantastic evening. The new decade (2010) dawns and life progresses as normal.

We manage to get in a fantastic skiing holiday in the Austrian/Italian Tyrol for a week in the Easter holidays with the Darnell family. I continue to attend my breast care groups, teach full time and work on my masters. Marcus has now taken up swimming and attends various galas. Lizzie starts taking her first GCSE exams in maths.

The Hatch End Triathlon comes round again, but this year I am not fit. I have a hip problem. I bet you are thinking, *oh for goodness sake, what else can go wrong with a body?* Well, it seems to me that what my mum told me was right. Getting old is horrible. My mind is writing cheques that my body can no longer afford to cash. My hip has actually been bothering me since last November and it is getting to the stage where I cannot walk without limping. I have been having regular osteopathic treatments, which helps, but of course friends immediately worry and want you to get it checked out in case it is something serious like cancer again.

So after some nagging, I go and see Sean Malloy again. In fact I see him the same day I see Adam Searle for my pre-operation planning meeting. Sean sends me for an MRI on my hip and fits me in at 7.20am in the morning for an appointment the following week to get the results. As it turns out there is something on the scan, but as Sean is not a hip specialist, he refers me to Matthew Bartlett. Clarifying that there is no bone cancer causing the pain means that the problem with my hip can go on the back burner till after I have reconstructive surgery, which is after all my main priority at the moment. However, it does mean no triathlon for me and in fact no running any more. I need to rethink my athletic regime in order to help combat the weight gain driven by the Tamoxifen.

The meeting with Adam goes very well and he mentally prepares me for what is to come. He explains exactly what he will do, how long it will take and what my recovery process will be like. This is it. I am actually going to do this. I am going to get a new breast. I am going to be a normal woman again phsyically. It is only as these thoughts go through my head that I realise I have just been in limbo for the last few months, mentally preparing myself for this phase of my treatment. Even though reconstructive surgery is not a treatment for cancer, it is a treatment that is required as a result of having had cancer. Therefore, strange though it may seem, psychologically it is inexplicably tied together with, how you cope with having had the disease.

Just before summer half term and a couple of weeks before the surgery, I have to go to the Royal Marsden to have all my pre-operative tests. I have an appointment and don't have to wait too

I FELT A RIGHT ONE...

long. I register all my insurance details and then see a very nice Canadian nurse. She spends a good hour going through my medical history incredibly thoroughly, weighs and measures me, checks my heart with an ECG and asks if I would mind having some photos taken before the surgery, as they like to keep a record of the benefit that they have made for patients. We also discuss the fact that I need to have a blood thinning injection in my stomach the evening before the surgery. As one of the side effects of Tamoxifen is DVT, which is caused by your blood becoming thicker, you need to have these injections to reduce this risk during surgery. The nurse asks if there is someone I can get to give me the injection and I call Sarah and Zoe, but neither are going to be available that evening. I ask if I can do it myself. How difficult can it be? People give themselves injections all the time for diabetes, fertility treatment and the like. I am, after all, only going to have to give myself one. I will need to collect the pre-prepared syringe the day before the surgery, which I can do when I come up for some final tests. The physiotherapist also comes to see me to prepare me for what she is going to want me to do and gives me a booklet to read on all the exercises that I am going to be expected to do each day following the surgery.

When all the preparations are complete and I have been fully briefed, I am given directions to the photographic department to get my pre-operation photos taken. I weave my way round the labyrinthine corridors in the basement to find the relevant department. A chap comes in, asks to see my permission form and again asks me all the questions about being photographed practically naked and do I mind that is by a male photographer. To be honest, I really have no modesty left any more. So many people have seen various parts of my anatomy naked, both male and female, that I really don't mind. When it is medically related, to them you are just a subject, like a piece of meat to be examined and analysed. There is nothing remotely sexual or inappropriate about their behaviour. They are incredibly professional and do absolutely everything they can to make you feel at ease, normally by chatting or giving you

Planning

instructions as to what you should be doing. I have great admiration for all the staff that have to deal with such personal issues of other people, like me.

I do think that hospitals should perhaps think more carefully about where they locate such a photography department. Yes, I know that in the basement there are no windows to cover up, but to the patient, it might make it feel a little seedy and down market. I am sure also that the staff may feel slightly unimportant in such a location, where in fact, visually recording the progress that patients make is something to celebrate and promote rather than tuck away in the basement. The photos take five minutes and then I wend my way out of the basement and back up to the daylight to get the tube home.

The day before the surgery, I have to have a procedure called a CT Angiogram. This is basically a scan of my abdomen, where they inject what is called a 'contrast medium', which allows the doctors to find all my blood vessels. This scan will help Adam Searle and his team identify where they are going to take the best blood vessels that supply the area of fat that they are going to use for the transplant to my chest.

A radiographer shows me into the scanner room. She explains that the only thing to be aware of is that when she gives me the injection of the dye, it might make me feel like I am weeing myself. I am so glad she tells me this, as it is the most extraordinary sensation and I really would have thought that I was wetting myself – all in all not a completely pleasant experience. However, it was over in less than five minutes and it means that the doctors have their roadmap to finding the best fat they can!

I walk round to the admissions department, where I had been told to go to collect my blood thinner to inject, only to discover it has not been prepared. I wait for an hour or so till Pauline, a sister on Adam Searle's plastic surgery team, comes to see me. She has been trying to phone me all day and she briefs me about what to make sure I bring into hospital with me – most importantly some soft bras with bra extenders. Luckily I already have these, as I would not have time to get them before tomorrow morning. I go down to the pharmacy and wait another forty five minutes or so. I finally get my prescription and get the train home.

Later that afternoon, one of my neighbours comes to see me. Another neighbour of ours died only a few days ago and the funeral is going to be on Monday morning and I will not be able to attend. June is also having a small operation tomorrow (Friday) and we talk about what had happened to Jenny, our friend and neighbour. Jenny had, about four weeks ago, gone into hospital for a commonplace operation. It seems anything that could go wrong did, and four weeks later she was dead – a real tragedy and not her time to go. I will miss her as both a neighbour and an immensely socially conscious member of our local community. She was a real pillar and performed many important formal roles on local committees. She will be missed very much. Hearing how things can go horribly wrong after such a regular operation is not really what I want to hear the day before undergoing a much more lengthy procedure. I cry for Jenny that evening, as it is truly a tragedy to lose such a kind and generous person in such an unfortunate way. It does make you realise that when your time is up, it is up and really there is not too much you can do about it. I am not exactly a fatalist, but I do believe that most things happen for a reason. We just don't always understand that reason, when we most feel we would like to understand it. Very often the reason is revealed to us when we least expect it, but nevertheless there is always a reason.

That evening at about 7pm I take myself off to the bedroom to inject myself. I have read the instructions carefully and set everything out on the bed ready. I asked Lizzie if she would like to watch, which she did and in fact I am glad she is there. Funnily enough, my bravado at saying I would be able to inject myself may have been a little optimistic. When actually holding the syringe, I completely balk at stabbing myself in the stomach. Lizzie has a great idea and suggests that I carefully grab the skin and fat, place the needle against the skin and push, she will then tell me when it is in far enough and I can then depress the plunger and inject the drug. This is what we do and I am so grateful that she is there to help me. I really don't think I could have done it on my own. Whilst upstairs I pack my bag ready; knickers, several pairs of pyjamas that have button-down-the-front tops, so that they are easy to put on and take off, wash bag, soft bras and bra extenders, mobile phone charger, a couple of books, slippers, a light dressing gown, an exercise booklet from the physio and finally my orthopaedic pillow.

I have a long, luxurious bath and generally enjoy the last bath that I am going to be able to have for the next six weeks or so. It may even be a few days till I can take a shower, so I really enjoy soaking like a whale for half an hour or so. I am not allowed to eat after 10pm that evening and not to drink past midnight. Pauline had told me that I can take small sips of water in the morning if I am really thirsty, as keeping hydrated is really important. I give both the children a big hug before they go to bed that night and tell them I will see them in hospital, probably on Saturday.

John and I go to bed early as we have to be up at 5.30am to get sorted, before we catch the train just after 6.00am at Harrow and Wealdstone Station in the morning. Of course getting to sleep is difficult. Everything runs through your mind, what might go wrong and how you are going to feel? You question again if you are doing the right thing and again I feel unutterably selfish for putting my family through this.

CHAPTER 21

They Can Rebuild You, they Have the Technology

I am of course totally awake before the alarm, get up and have a quick shower and wash my hair. Hairdresser friend, Karen, had been only the week before and I have gone as short as I dare, just so it's easier to take care of whilst I am not too mobile. The children know we won't be there when they get up, but Lizzie did ask that I go in and give her a kiss before I leave. I cannot help myself and go in and give them both one before I go.

We catch the tube to South Kensington and walk the short, pleasant walk through the Chelsea side streets, assessing the parking metre situation for when John will have to drive up and bring me home. We go through the main entrance and wait along with several other people who are obviously also there for surgery that day. Why else would anyone be there at such an ungodly hour?

We arrive at about 7.10am and so are early then after only five minutes waiting, the fire alarm goes off! We are asked to move down the corridor until we can no longer hear the alarm and wait. Someone will come back and get us when we are allowed. Another little bit of background here. About eighteen to twenty-four months ago the Royal Marsden suffered a major fire and in fact the rebuilding works are still going on. This, I am sure, makes them understandably a little paranoid about fire alarms. Apparently they go off with monotonous regularity, which must drive the poor staff totally mad, as how do you know if it is real or not?

John and I move around to the side of the hospital and John pops back every few minutes to see if the alarm has stopped. We wait by the pharmacy (at least I now know my way round the hospital, which is helpful in this situation) and then go to the outpatients reception, where there is a small coffee shop. John gets a coffee and we go outside and walk round to the front of the hospital to the main entrance where we see the firemen getting back into their engines. We walk back to the front door and are told we can come back in. It is now gone 7.30 and I hope this is not going to delay us for too long as I just want to get on with it.

About five minutes later my name is called and we are taken up to the operating theatre booking-in department. The staff had been kept in during the alarm, but had not been allowed downstairs to get us whilst the alarm was on. Another five minutes passes and then my admissions nurse calls my name and takes me through to a curtained area, where there are several other patients being taken through the same booking-in process as me.

The petite, middle aged, Spanish nurse attaches a plastic name bracelet to both my right arm and leg. She also attaches another which highlights an allergy – for me, elastoplast and some other forms of sticking plaster. She goes through a detailed pre-operative checklist, asking most of the questions I had been asked two weeks ago, but it is reassuringly thorough. By now it is just past 8.00am. She gives me a gown and says I can keep my own cotton knickers on as they are going to take them off in theatre anyway. I get some blue foam, disposable slippers and put on a full length set of compression stockings. These are particularly fetching and have some sort of semi-adhesive rubber nodules at the top to stop them slipping down!

The nurse keeps getting interrupted by doctors throughout this process. First it is Adam and two colleagues. John and I are introduced to both of them and then he gets down to business with his measuring tape and magic marker. He is discussing with Charlie, his registrar, what he is planning to do, asking him what he thinks. I ask what order he will do things. He says he will start off by working on the reduction of the left breast first and then will work on harvesting the fat and skin tissue from my belly. He will then be working on the vascular part of the transplant whilst Charlie tidies up the lower part of my abdomen.

Adam uses what can only be described as a dress makers measuring tape. I start to giggle to myself and John looks at me quizzically. I say to the assembled group, "You know, I feel just like something out of a Hannibal Lecter film, like you are measuring my skin up to use bits to make a body suit for someone else!"

John smiles, knowing that I am using my humour to diffuse what he can see for me is quite a nerve racking situation.

As I look down at all the measurements, markings and arrows he is drawing on me, I ask the question, "OK then, tell me, how on earth do you guys actually work out what things are going to look like after the surgery – how much fat do you know how to take and what shape the breast will finally be when all the swelling dies down and it settles into its final resting place?"

Charlie, quick as a flash responds with, "Optimistic patients and lax ethics committees!"

We all laugh out loud and I start to feel more relaxed. Adam takes about ten minutes all in all and is gentle, supportive, relaxed and positive all the way through.

I wonder what it must feel like for poor John at this time, watching me being drawn all over and talked about like a slab of meat. He seems to take it all in his stride, but I think it helps that Adam and his team talk to him as well, not just me. They recognise the importance the partner has to play in all of this and do not ignore him in any way. It shows me that they really do understand the psychological processes that a couple must go through and not just the patient alone.

When Adam is finished he gives me a big smile and tells me I will see him after the surgery. The nurse comes back and carries on with the checklist. The next interruption is from David, the anaesthetist. He is really important in this operation as it is so long – anywhere between six to ten hours. My biggest worry is what pain relief he will use. I know now that morphine makes me incredibly ill, having had two surgeries where I had morphine, my mastectomy and having the disc out of my neck in 1997. We discuss this and he comes up with an alternative that he can use. He asks about teeth etc, in case I swallow any during the operation and choke! I also tell him about the fact that my left eye does not react to light in the normal way, in fact the pupil gets smaller when it gets dark and gets larger when light is shined into it, a condition I have had for a few years. Not normally a problem, unless some unknowing doctor or nurse shines a light into your eye to check the status of your brain, gets an unusual response and panics as a result. You really don't want to be thought to have something wrong with your brain when you are not awake to tell them that you are really perfectly fine! We also talk about my sticking plaster allergy and he plans to use nothing that should affect me. Good.

Our discussion takes about five minutes and when he is satisfied he says he will see me downstairs in a few minutes. The nurse comes back, finishes off and then tells me it is time to go down to theatre. I give my watch and everything else to John, except my glasses. I give him a big hug and kiss and tell him I will see him when I wake up. This is it, time to go. When I next see John I will be a new woman, literally!

He is going to take my bag and put it in a locker and then go home till early afternoon. There is no point in him sitting around the hospital all day, he may as well go home and sort things out (I think he secretly wants to check I have not put sand in the bed this time!) I also know that he will be entertained as today, is the opening day of the World Cup in South Africa. I could not have chosen a better time to have the operation, as whilst John has some time off work, he can also watch the footie!

I FELT A RIGHT ONE...

The nurse walks me down to theatre. You can tell that there are building works going on as we pass lots of workmen and the theatre suite is not as organised as I am sure it would normally be. I sit on a chair outside the theatre doors whilst the nurse passes responsibility for me over to the theatre sister. She is very thorough and will not let me out of her hands until she has the correct signatures and paper work. I am then shown into the operating room. I hand my glasses to the nurse, who puts them with my dressing gown and slippers.

David, the anaesthetist, is there with his colleague. It takes two of them for such a long operation and with so much going on. I get up onto the operating table, which has some soft gel padding on it to reduce the likelihood of pressure sores, as I will be lying still in the same position for quite a long time. As I am going to be on the table for several hours they take a lot of care to make sure that I am as comfortable as I can be. My arms have to be held in place in arm rests and all the needles have to go into my left hand. They will be inserting a catheter into my urethra so that I don't have to worry about weeing for a while – a relief to me, as I remember the difficulties that I had last time. It takes David a little while to decide which veins to use for the cannulas. The problem with having had your lymph nodes removed in one arm and chemotherapy in the other one is that you cannot use the veins in the side with the lymph nodes removed and the ones you are left with are very difficult to use. From the patient's perspective, this means that any blood tests or cannulas in the future are more painful than they were before and often means more than one try is made due to the difficulty of finding good enough veins – so again, more pain.

Please don't think I'm moaning, as you learn to take things like this in your stride. I hope that anyone reading this might now see the broader range of impacts that cancer treatment has on a person. These things force the patient to remember their cancer, even when they may wish to totally forget about it after coming out the other side.

When everything is in place and I am as comfortable as I am going to be for some time to come, David asks if I am ready and tells me it is time to put me to sleep. As he is injecting the anaesthetic he talks to me gently, telling me the sensations I should be feeling. *This is it*, I think as I drift off, *when I wake up I will…*

The next thing I know, I am drowsily returning to consciousness in a completely different place. The first thing I do is ask for John. When I open my eyes again he is sitting next to me. I ask the time and it is about 5.00pm. The whole day has gone – all in all the operation took about seven hours. I now have a chance to take a look at myself for the first time since coming into the recovery room. Well, actually it is the High Dependency Unit (HDU), as after such a long anaesthetic I think you are a higher risk and so they keep an extra eye on you for a while. I am feeling remarkably good. Drugs are wonderful when you really need them. I feel no pain and am still so high I cannot really feel how hot I actually am.

Let's explain the details here. I am in a bed attached to a whole host of wires, tubes and other equipment. Firstly the catheter, so I can wee. Then the five drains which capture any excess blood and serous fluid which the wounds secrete internally after the surgery. There are two in my groin area, two under my right arm on the side of the transplant and one of the left side for the reduction. Next, each leg has a massager on it, which slowly inflates and deflates a cuff around each of my calves in turn, to make sure that the blood is circulating properly. Two drips in my left hand, one to deliver fluids and the other with the Patient Controlled Analgesia (PCA), which is the pain relief that I can request when I feel I need it. Because of this pain relief, an oxygen mask is needed because the pain medication lowers your natural respiration rate and you are at risk of reduced blood oxygen levels. Last but not least, the Bair Hugger. This is a blanket made up of pockets of warm air provided by a heated air pump at the bottom of the bed. This is really important as my body temperature must be kept above normal. The doctors want the capillaries, the smallest of blood vessels, to remain as open as possible to make sure that there is a good blood flow to all the skin in the transplant to increase the rate of healing. It also keeps the bigger blood vessels wider, which reduces the strain on the transplanted veins and arteries and particularly on the join. It is this join which is at risk of failure.

Quite soon after I wake up, I get taken down to the ward where I am going to spend my time recuperating. It seems a long way through the ward, past individual rooms and four bed bays, round the corner, right to the end. I am put in a strange shaped room, which turns out to be one that is specially designed for patients who receive internal radiotherapy and have to be kept isolated. I am tucked in round the corner.

I am very tired but very excited and not really in any pain – just extremely hot and very sweaty! I now get a chance to take a look at my chest. I peer down and carefully lift the top edge of my very fetching hospital gown to have a look. I have a noticeable cleavage! I start to smile and in fact the smile does not leave my face for several weeks. I have a new breast and, wow, it is great. I am so amazed at how high up the tissue comes under the skin of my chest. It has filled up the concave void which showed my top two ribs on the right-hand side of my chest. Great! I had no idea that I would be so pleased – I am ecstatic and I am experiencing a total and complete psychological high, which I am sure also helps anaesthetise any pain I am supposed to feel.

I look at John and he smiles back at me. I think perhaps he now realises that having the mastectomy may have affected me more than even he had thought. I certainly realise that it must have affected me at a subliminal level. Maybe I had just not let it bother me. After all what was the point, I couldn't do anything about it, could I? What is the point in being negative and fed up about something that you cannot actually change. Yes, I know that everyone is different, but I have through the whole of my life really tried to live by this maxim. I have really achieved something by not letting having only one breast bother me. But now, wow, I am really going to enjoy having one back again! It is not yet perfect, but it is so much better than none at all. In fact even less than none due to the indentation it had left at the top of my chest, which you would not normally think of as breast tissue, but which actually is.

David pops in to check I am OK and to find out about how the pain is. I am honestly able to tell him that I don't feel sick and that I am actually not in as much pain as I thought I would be. He is very happy, bids John and I farewell and leaves.

I now get to meet Margaret, the sweet nurse assigned to me for the next twelve hours or so. It is going to be her job to sit with me and check the transplant every quarter of an hour to start with. After four hours or so it will reduce to half an hour, then after another four hours it will drop to hourly and then after that every two hours. This time is extremely crucial, as it is the most likely time that anything will go wrong. The most common part to fail is where the blood vessels have been joined in at the chest. If this happens, I will have to have immediate surgery again to repair it. The chances are slim, but they take the precaution of allocating a specific nurse, just to look out for this. I am incredibly impressed.

By now, John is getting tired and he needs to go home and sort the children out. He bids me farewell and tells me he will be up tomorrow morning. Marcus has football, but he will bring Lizzie up with him. I am brought a really light dinner, which I am decidedly ready for and eat a little bit. All the while, Margaret sits and knits.

Not long after John left, Adam Searle arrives to see how I am. He must be totally shattered, but is dressed smartly again and looks ready for a night out on the town. How do they do it? Work a twelve hour day, most of it on their feet, working with such intensity and then still have the energy to come and see you to make sure you are OK. Adam makes me laugh when he tells me that earlier this morning, whilst I was down in theatre with the anaesthetists, he was in the canteen with Charlie and Pauline stocking up on food in readiness for this marathon of an operation, when John comes up to him and says, "Aren't you supposed to be cutting my wife open right now?"

Apparently he responded with, "Well you wouldn't want me and my team to work on your wife for so long on an empty stomach now, would you?"

I can just imagine Johnny doing it, which makes me giggle. Adam is sorry that he did not get up to see me earlier whilst John was with me, but tells me he is really pleased with how the operation went. He has a look at his handiwork and shows Margaret exactly where she needs to test the pulse. He has placed a tiny stitch on the surface of the skin to indicate where the best place to hear the blood flow is. Margaret will have to use a small electronic listening device to hear the pulse. When she tests it I can hear the reassuring beat of my heart pumping blood through my new breast tissue. It is really quite thrilling and very emotional; it is concrete evidence that I have a new part to my body that is totally mine.

Adam looks at all the wounds and for the first time I get to see how flat my stomach is. Well, not totally, as he tells me there is quite a lot of swelling and that it can take three or four months, perhaps longer, for it to fully settle down to its natural state again. Wow, I can see parts of my body that I have not been able to see, except in a mirror, for a very long time, certainly not since having had the children!! I have a better figure than I did before and my smile gets even bigger, if that were possible. The wound from where they have removed the fat goes more than half way round my body, from hip to hip. It dips down at the front and sits just above my pubic hair. I look like I have been bitten by a shark! There is no other way to describe it.

Adam points out where all the drains are and I ask how long they will have to stay in. He comments that everyone is individual, but that they will take them out as soon as they are not draining so much fluid – apparently 40ml per twenty-four hour period. The nurses will record the figure each day and then a decision can be made. He checks all my charts and when he is totally sure that I am fine he tells me he will be back to see me in the morning. After he leaves I feel totally exhausted and know it is time to rest. Margaret tells me to just put my head down, to use the PCA if I need it and that she will try to be as gentle as possible when she has to check the flap – not an attractive name for a transplant, but then most medical terms are pretty unpleasant.

The night passes in a blur really, but I do get a pretty good night's sleep, all things considered. I know that Margaret keeps coming over, lifting the Bair Hugger cover off and carefully lifting the bedclothes and my gown to get at the listening site, but she is so gentle that I don't really notice it most of the time. It is as if my body knows that sleep is the best thing for me and makes sure I get it. There are the normal observations as well, but as I have the PCA to give myself pain drugs if I need them I won't really get disturbed until the morning drugs round. I know that they will not take the oxygen mask off until I stop using the PCA and actually I am not really in that much pain. I take as little as I can and still manage some reasonable sleep.

In no time at all it is the morning and Adam is back to see how I am getting on. Margaret says I am doing amazingly well, she tells me that she has sat with very many patients like me and that I had the best night's sleep with as little pain relief as she had ever seen. This is a real boost mentally as it reinforces what I already feel, which is that I cannot believe I have undergone a seven hour surgery.

Adam, delighted with how everything is going, also comments that some of the drainage bottles don't seem to be receiving much fluid, so there is a chance that some of the drains may come out tomorrow. Yippee!

You know I think spending time in hospital, especially when so restricted by medical equipment, is a bit like being in the Big Brother House. You are focused on such small issues which in the outside world would seem insignificant, but for the time you are there, this is your whole world, your whole universe in fact and so each tiny activity, target, test, seems to take on an overly large importance.

I FELT A RIGHT ONE...

I now discover that Adam and his family live in the country and that during the week he stays in London, returning home to be with his family for the weekend. He feels I am well enough that he can return home. This again I take as a good sign, as I trust him implicitly and know that he would not take any risks with my care. He must be feeling really confident with his handiwork to make that decision. He gives me both his home phone number and his mobile number, in case I have any worries at all and feel the need to speak to him. He tells me that it is fine to call him at home as his wife is also a doctor and totally understands.

He leaves and then the routine of the hospital day starts. Margaret has literally nursed me through the most crucial part of the recovery and has been a real delight to be with. It makes me realise that nursing for most people truly is a vocation and that to be on the receiving end of such care is actually a privilege. It is now time for her to take her leave. She has performed her crucial duty of ensuring that all Adam and his team's hard work has not gone to waste, by making sure that the transplant is working properly. She packs up her knitting, bids me farewell and leaves me to the care of the normal ward staff.

CHAPTER 22

I Can Feel a Right One Again

John and Lizzie come to visit at about 10.00am and I am so pleased to see them. Lizzie is fascinated by all the equipment and asks lots of intelligent questions about what everything is and what it does. I tell Lizzie what Margaret had said about how well I was doing with pain relief and sleep and she exclaims, "Mum you are so competitive, I can't believe that you would want to have taken the least pain relief, are you mad?"

I honestly never thought I would be pleased to say it, but it is good having a catheter! The thought of actually moving out of bed to go to the loo is too frightening to think about. Hopefully if some of the drains come out tomorrow then I can also get rid of some of the other contraptions, including the bag! I am also sweating so much that I can feel it dripping down my new cleavage. So a good thing really! I am desperate for a shower or wash of some sort. The nurses realise this and very kindly give me a bed bath after John and Lizzie have left.

In the afternoon, John comes back with Marcus and Lizzie. Visitors are great as they make the time pass more quickly and even though you can get tired there is enough time to rest in between. I mention to Lizzie that my hair feels horrible and she offers to wash it for me tomorrow so I know I might start to look a little more presentable.

Now there is only one problem with the room that I am in, which is that the television does not work. Apparently, when they were undergoing the refurbishment work after the fire, the cable got messed up and they have not had a chance to sort it out yet. John had brought in a portable ariel to see if that would help, but as the room is lead lined, not a chance! So instead of watching television I read lots of books, as well as dozing and resting.

On the Sunday morning, Adam Searle phones in from home to see if I am OK. I speak to him and he reminds me to tell the nurses about a stitch that is holding one of the drains in place so that it does not hurt as much when they take it out. He has chatted to the nurses and they are going to take out three of the drains, which is great. I can also have the leg pumps removed and the catheter, so that I can get up and start to move around.

After his call, Lisa, one of the nurses, gets everything ready to remove the catheter and the drains. She and another nurse work together and even though it is a relief to have the them removed, it is a really weird sensation to have some tubing (up to 20cm of it) pulled out of various parts of your body. The only drains I am left with are the two in my groin, to keep the swelling down in the area where the fat was taken from. One of the cannulas had been removed this morning, so now I just have to carry my two drain bottles and be careful with my left hand, but I can get up and go to the loo myself. Hurrah!

That afternoon, I actually get up and walk very carefully to the little bathroom. I have been warned that you need to try and stand as upright as you can, as the temptation is to hunch over to protect your stomach. Again it is a very strange sensation and the skin feels very tight, which of course it is. I can make it to an almost upright position and am really pleased with myself. I am even able to walk down the corridor. Lizzie manages to wash my hair over the sink and I feel human again. I have given myself a body wash, used the bidet and got clean hair. What more can a girl ask for?

I actually have quite a lot of visitors over the few days I am in,

I Can Feel a Right One Again

for which I am very grateful. They have all left by 8.00pm and I settle down with a book and get a good night's sleep.

On Monday morning Charlie, Adam's Registrar, comes round to see me and is very impressed with my progress. The drains in my groin are still collecting quite a lot of fluid, and he reinforces that I cannot go home until there is less than 40ml per twenty-four hour period. I say thank you to him for all his hard work on getting my body back to normality and find myself getting very emotional about it. I am very teary. I am sure some of the emotion that I am exhibiting is just a release, from both the stress of the surgery and the after effects of the rather long anaesthetic, but also just because it is part of the mental healing process. This surgery and whatever comes after it are part of the whole recovery process from having had cancer. This is the first major step in getting my body back to a more natural shape. When my body feels more normal, I will be more able to forget what has happened to me and think to the future rather than the past. Charlie seems to understand my need for emotional release, but thanks me for what I have said.

Adam also drops by fairly early and is really pleased with my progress. Seeing how happy Charlie and Adam are with the way I am healing and getting on gives me a real psychological boost. I know all my friends worry that I am a bit pig-headed and that I am at risk of overdoing things too quickly, but these doctors' reassurances have shown me that you can do difficult things. I know my own body, my own pain and energy thresholds and am also a very determined and driven person. I want to get home to my own, comfortable bed as soon as possible. Although the Royal Marsden is a wonderful place, it is not the easiest place to get to from Harrow for people to visit. The sooner I get home, the easier it will be for everyone.

Adam briefs me on the fact that I now need to get some supportive knickers! I laugh out loud, "Like Bridget Jones?" I ask with a smile.

"Absolutely!" responds Adam, but in a slightly more serious tone explains how "they will help reduce the swelling and protect the wound." He looks at the sports bra's I have bought in and says I need to start wearing one all the time, even in bed for a few weeks. We discuss how long I will have to stay in hospital and he says he feels that I can probably go home on Wednesday, even with one drain left in. He arranges for one more drain to be taken out today. He tells me he will be back tomorrow and off he goes.

Each day I am in hospital I have to have a blood thinning injection to counteract the effects of Tamoxifen. The irony is that the site where the injection is given always comes up in a big bruise. I have blood tests, which the nurse finds hard to get, surprise, surprise. I am now only taking paracetamol and Diclofenac (painkiller and anti-inflammatory), as well as antibiotics.

Sarah comes to see me this morning and I show her how well I am doing by getting up and walking up and down the corridor. Whilst she is there the physio pops in to check up on me. Her only concern is whether I can manage stairs, as I need to be able to do that before I can go home. I am totally up for it and suggest that we go and try some stairs now. Sarah joins us and I get my first walk out of the ward since I have come out of surgery. I feel like a prisoner let out of their cell for a while. It is marvellous. We make our way slowly to the main staircase, where I show how well I can already manage stairs. The physio is very happy with me, checks how I am getting on with the exercises and then says she is confident that I will be fine to go home whenever the doctors are ready to let me go.

Later in the afternoon, Annie Wheelie comes to see me on her way home from work (or rather after work and it is not really 'on her way'). She brings me some chocolate and marshmallows. I share the news that I will probably be home on Wednesday with everyone and phone Zoe to ask if she can procure me some large, but supportive knickers before she comes to see me tomorrow.

On Tuesday, I feel the dressings start to itch. I am quite allergic to a whole range of sticking plasters and it seems that what they have used on me is no exception. The fact that it is so warm, I am sure, makes it worse. Zoe comes in to see me in the morning and whilst she is with me, Pauline the plastic surgery sister comes in to see me. She is going to change all my dressings and hopefully reduce the amount of plaster stuck to my skin, which should reduce the irritation.

As Zoe was a nurse and as I am happy with it, she can stay while Pauline does all the work. We are all chatting away, when there is a knock on the door. "Come in," I call out.

"Hang on a second," says Pauline loudly, "who is it?"

"The cleaner," comes the reply.

"Would you mind coming back later as I am just working with the patient," responds Pauline, quickly.

"What are you like?" Zoe comments. "Had you forgotten that you are practically naked, when you told them to 'come in'?"

"Well, actually, I had!" I laughed. It just goes to show you that you become so used to exposing your body all the time and so many people taking a look, that even when a total stranger knocks on the door I forget that I should probably not say 'come in'. The three of us laugh about it, but I must remember to be slightly more circumspect in future.

Zoe has brought with her a range of underwear for me, in readiness for going home. It is so sweet of her to have spent the time to go shopping for me and I am so grateful. Not long after she leaves, another friend arrives. Lisa is over from the US and has managed to find the time to come and see me. I am so touched. She stays for about an hour and is on her way back to the States, having spent a week or so in Europe. I have not seen her for a couple of years since she returned home and it is good to catch up and hear all about her new life in Dallas. We chat about mutual friends. How kind that she found time in her busy schedule to come and visit me. I know she has a soft spot for the Royal Marsden as she held a house clearance sale before she returned to America and all the proceeds were donated to the hospital.

I FELT A RIGHT ONE...

That evening John comes up with the children for one final visit before I come home tomorrow. Whilst they are here, Simone also comes to see me. She has driven in from Hounslow where she teaches and she offers to drive John and the kids home. They decline and in fact she stays chatting till nearly 10.00pm. Poor Simone, she is going to be so tired at school tomorrow.

On Wednesday morning John arrives at about 10.00am and we just have to wait around to be briefed on what to do when I go home. Adam comes to see me whilst John is there and he sees me dressed and ready to go. He is very pleased with how I look in clothes and so am I.

I turn to him to thank him and again feel myself welling up with emotion. I try to explain how I feel, but he already knows. He must have seen this so many times and clearly understands the enormous emotional impact that something like reconstructive surgery has on people. Having this kind of surgery has made me rethink my view on cosmetic surgery as a whole. I think I have been quite judgemental about people wanting look a certain way and I still do find it sad that society is such (through the influence of the media) that individuals feel they can only achieve happiness through significant physical changes. However, having this operation has made me reconsider my views.

Who am I to judge other people? If I felt so driven to have reconstructive surgery even before I had my mastectomy, so why shouldn't anyone have something done that is going to make them feel better about themselves and improve their self-esteem? People choose to have cosmetic surgery for all sorts of reasons and are my reasons any better or worse than theirs? OK, so I had cancer and if you like, this process I am going through is a by-product of that – cause and effect.

I guess part of my brain still wonders why anyone would put themselves through surgery when they don't have to, but I didn't have to either. My operation was not a matter of life or death; it was just to make me feel psychologically better. So, ultimately, I am no different to anyone else. I have felt the hugely beneficial mental boost that I have received, even whilst still in hospital, so imagine how I am going to feel in a few weeks time when everything has settled down?

It just goes to show you that every life experience, either positive or negative, is a learning experience and if you take the time to think carefully about the impact of any experience, you can normally work something out about yourself that you may not have realised before. John always tells me I over-think things and perhaps I do, but as I get older I am not so sure that it is such a bad thing. I no longer try to worry about things I cannot affect, but to invest time and examine what makes you tick is well worth the effort.

I know that I still open my mouth before I have engaged my brain, more than I would like, but I feel I understand my reaction to others and their reactions to me, much more clearly than I did before I got sick. Another significant silver lining from that big old cloud.

By about 11.00ish, all my papers and medicines are ready and I can leave. Pauline has given me a little handmade bag to carry my drain around in. It is like having a small pet permanently attached! I will need to phone each day to give the amount of fluid that has been drained and then they will let me know when I need to come back in to have it removed. I cannot wait as the stitch that holds the tube in place, just above my pubic hair, pulls any time the tube gets caught on something, or moves against the top of my knickers. It is generally annoying, but better this than staying in till I stop producing fluid.

John has taken one load of stuff to the car and just needs to carry the last bits and act as my guard dog as I walk out. On the ground floor, as we are leaving the hospital, there is a book sale on and I cannot resist having a look. John is a little exasperated, but I assure him that a little retail therapy is just what I need, especially after five days on my own in a room without a TV! I make a few purchases to add to the present cupboard at home and then finally we are off. It

I FELT A RIGHT ONE...

is only a short walk to the car and John has brought up some towels for me to fold over and act as padding between my wounds and the seat belt. We slowly wend our way out through the London traffic and make our way home. Wow, it is good to be outside in the fresh air, well almost fresh! I am so looking forward to being home and back to some level of normality.

When we get home, I am shattered and go upstairs to have a lie down. Basically, I just rest, watch TV, read and start to think about my masters degree work that needs to be done. The next day, I send out an email:

Email sent out on 17.6.10 entitled – I feel a right one again.

Dear Friends
    For those of you that don't know and I know many do, I have just got out of hospital after having reconstructive surgery.
    Yes, believe it or not they can rebuild you! After many generous offers of fat donations from other people, I rightly decided that it would be best if I used my own (I did have rather a lot to spare, it has to be said). Anyway seven hours of surgery, being connected to eleven different things on the bed for the first thirty-six hours and five days in hospital later, I am home. I still have a drain in, but with luck that will come out tomorrow.
    On Saturday morning, whilst being cooked nicely under what is fondly called a 'Bair Hugger' which basically blows warm air into a blanket to keep all the blood vessels open and working; with five drains, two drug drips, oxygen and two leg massage pumps (which may sound nice but with nylon tight stockings underneath and sweating profusely is a little annoying), I really did think to myself "what the f*** have I done?" Carrying a kilo of silicone (looking like a large turkey fillet) around in a bra was not such a bad thing, was it?
    Anyway six days later and although looking like I have been beaten up by Frank Bruno (body, not face) I am amazed at what

medical science can do! I realise how lucky I am to have received such truly amazing medical care. Believe it or not, I did not have enough fat to make a G cup breast. Surely not! I hear you say. So they also had to make my left one smaller. On Friday morning whilst being marked up with a permanent marker by the plastic surgeon, I did say to him at the time that it felt like being measured by Hannibal Lecter and that my skin could be used to make a body suit for someone. At this point I think he realised the depravity of my sense of humour! So they had already done a CT Angiogram of my abdomen which shows them where the good veins and arteries are and also they are planning where to take the fat from. The size of my new right one is going to be determined by the area of fat one vein and artery can supply. Definitely not enough for a G cup, but perhaps enough for a C?

So, with stitches from hip to hip, a smaller left one (which will still shrink a bit due to swelling) and a completely new right one (less nipple!) I am 80% there. The amazing thing is that where my chest was all hollowed out from the mastectomy, the surgical team have been able to fill it back out, so with clothes I look fine. I now have no belly and my navel has been relocated in the skin that was pulled down. Sorry for those of you that did not want to know the graphic detail; however, you just have to understand how amazing it all really is. My new right one, with the assistance of gravity, will drop to a similar level as the left one over the next few months and then I just have to go for some tidying up over the next year. A bit of liposuction to get rid of the 'dog ears' (technical plastic surgery term!) at my sides, perhaps have a new nipple built and an areola tattooed and I will be as good as new.

Adam, the surgeon, said the first step is to look good in normal clothes (and girls out there, I am up for a new wardrobe with my smaller chest!) then in a swimsuit, and then finally naked. I cannot express the positive psychological benefit. It is amazing. I had thought I didn't care about not having a right one and that it was just the inconvenience of carrying a very uncomfortable amount of silicone around every day, which I am sure is a large part of it. But to feel that actually I am going to have a better body than I started with two years ago, gives quite a positive mental boost. Now don't get me wrong, I am not saying that I would ever have wanted to have had breast cancer in the first place, but it just shows you that truly every cloud has a silver lining. Johnny gets a forty-eight year old wife with a thirty year old's body!!

I have to say thank you to all my family and friends for letting me be so 'out there' with all that has happened to me, as I am sure you have not always wanted to hear what I felt I needed to say. I really do appreciate your willingness to listen and promise you that there is not too much more to come.

Come visit one and all, and stop me from getting too bored.

On Friday morning, John takes me back up to the Royal Marsden so that Pauline can take the final drain out and change my dressings. It is such a relief to be free. I wear loose clothes when possible, as it is so hot to wear the big knickers all the time! I do keep a bra on, but use a bra extender to make sure it is not too tight and digging into the stitches. It is amazing. There really are not too many stitches on the outside, most of them are internal. I am reliably informed that there are hundreds inside. Some of them, especially the knots, will take months to dissolve, possibly up to eight.

The following week I have a visit to the nurse to remove some stitches (where the drains were) and to check the wounds. I also go to see Adam so that he can check his handiwork. Generally he is pleased, but does comment that the left breast, which although he made smaller, in my eyes considerably so, will still need more adjustment.

You know, it is hard to believe that I actually did not have enough fat to make a breast as big as my remaining one. I had been trying, well not really trying, more not worrying, about my weight in preparation for this, as I knew I would need as much fat as I could get, but it still was not enough. My new breast is much more pert and sits slightly higher than the left one, and I can see that I am going to still need a little bit of stuffing in the right side of my bra to make things look even. Now I just need to wait for all the swelling to go down and then in six months or so we can consider the next stage.

Shortly after we get home from my check up, Stevi arrives from Dubai to stay for a couple of days. It is so nice just to spend time chatting and relaxing and we get a mutual friend over for lunch the next day. Stevi leaves on Thursday and then on Friday we go to Hatch End to see Lizzie performing in *Return to the Forbidden Planet*. It is a lot of fun and it is good to catch up with people.

I actually manage to walk up to school that week to take in my sick note and use the photocopier for some of my assignment work. It is tiring, but I do need to not be a couch potato or to wrap myself in cotton wool too much.

For the next month, my life is fairly quiet. However, I have now decided to write this book, but will not allow myself to start until I finish my 10,000 word master's assignment, so I get cracking on it. I have all the information I need, all the books and data, I just need to sit down and do the work.

I have a couple more visits to the see Kirsten the nurse at Adam Searle's consulting rooms and also see Adam again. During this time I find myself getting a little low and on one of my visits to see Kirsten I actually end up crying. She is brilliant and seems to understand what is going on, when I don't. Her experience with so many patients and life changing surgery has equipped her well enough to notice the emotional signals that we patients must emit.

I don't think it is the enormity of what I have been through, but the mundaneliness and length of time that you feel discomfort which can get you down. Wearing a bra is constantly uncomfortable and I guess I hadn't realised how strange my stomach would feel, or not feel as the case may be. It seems I am slowly increasing the amount of skin on my body which has no sensation because the nerves have been cut. I know it sounds like I am complaining, but I am not. For me, being normally so positive, I really don't like being down at all. I find it annoying and it makes me feel like I am not in control, but I do recognise the importance of the emotional release that crying gives and Kirsten is there to support me with her kind words and a gentle hug.

CHAPTER 23

Committing Pen to Paper

I get my 10,000 word assignment in on time and then treat myself to starting my book. I have been making notes, keeping them in a lovely book that one of my colleagues gave me for Christmas. It's from Paperchase – need I say more? I trawl through my email history, diary, calendar and photo archive. This gives me most of the factual and chronological information that I need.

It is an interesting experience to actually decide to write a book. I have never thought I could seriously have a go at such a significant undertaking. Do I even know enough words to put in a book? Jon Cobb, who I met through Hunty, was one of the people who emailed me when I first started telling a wider group of friends and had sent me a brilliantly written piece about his experiences when being treated for testicular cancer. It had me in hysterics and was so witty, punchy and used fantastic observational humour, that I felt motivated to try and replicate his efforts. My style is nowhere near as good as his, but it gave me the idea for my journal, which I had started keeping, and so I did not have to start from scratch.

For some reason, though, I am compelled to do it. It is another challenge and as you can already see, I do quite like those. I have decided that I would like, if possible, to try and get it published and that will be no tall order. If you are reading this now, then I have achieved my goal.

I FELT A RIGHT ONE...

I wonder if anyone will want to read it? Why am I writing it? Well, for several reasons. By taking the time to go through the last two years in detail, it allows me to closely analyse what I think and feel and why I think and feel it. I do feel a little self-absorbed or even narcissistic doing it, but the thought that if I can get it published I could actually make some money which can go to charity is a big motivator.

The thing is that so many men and women go through the same emotional and physical roller coaster that I have been on and I have not read any accounts that I found helped me to deal with what I had to go through. The breast support group at the hospital really helps and it is the understanding that you are not on your own and that other people know exactly how you feel that is really helpful. Not everyone, however, has the benefit of such a group.

I have been asked by a range of people to talk to other breast cancer sufferers, in particular about the experiences I have had, in order to support them through theirs. So perhaps there is an audience for a book that documents the whole range of physical, emotional and psychological processes that a cancer patient can go through.

Writing, I find, is a release. It allows me to really think and analyse my own thought processes relating to a whole range of issues. You don't really realise how momentous and life changing, suffering from such a significant disease is, until it happens. I have found that it is worth the investment of time and energy to carefully consider the specific impacts it has on you as a person.

I find myself really enjoying the process of writing, but realise that I probably could never write a work of fiction. The children I teach could definitely do a better job than me in that area. It seems I cannot imagine very well, but that observing reality and describing it seems to come more naturally to me.

Although I am signed off work until the middle of July, I do go into school and teach some sex and relationship education to year five and spend some time with my class before they leave for high school. I attend their graduation evening and their prom and although completely shattered afterwards, I am glad that I am actually able to go. I have spent so much time with these children and so enjoyed seeing them develop and grow as people. They have also been incredibly supportive to me. I want to give them a present for when they leave and I spend a few hours of the spare time I have making them each a book mark. When I was working part time I had attended calligraphy classes, so I put my skills to work and hand write their name in gold ink on black paper, sign the back of each one and laminate it. I take them in and give them out on the last day of school.

After term has finished, I spend a short time tidying and readying my classroom for the beginning of the next academic year and then time for the summer holidays.

CHAPTER 24

It's Only Pain

Now that things have settled down on the reconstructive process, it is time to get my hip sorted. My hip has been hurting more and more and I go to see Matthew Bartlett, as Sean Malloy has suggested. When I see him in early August, he tells me that I have some degeneration in the hip joint and that he can try to help the pain and discomfort with a cortisone injection. I have had several of these before in my Achilles tendons and in the soles of my feet. They are excruciatingly painful as I remember and the thought of one in my hip is not a pleasant one.

He tells me that he would give me the injection under general anaesthetic, in order to manage the potential pain. He discusses possible options if the injection doesn't work, which could be an arthroscopy or a hip replacement. Matthew is however very honest and says that although I have been referred to him and he does deal with hips, he is more a knee specialist. If I need more treatment later then he will refer me onto someone else who specialises in hips. We arrange that I will have the injection the following week. Again I am at the Clementine Churchill Hospital; a building I seem to have spent a lot of time in during the last couple of years.

The morning of my mini-operation, which is what it is as I have to have a general anaesthetic, I have the same anaesthetist who put me to sleep for my mastectomy. Furthermore, the nurse who greets me down at theatre is none other than Cleo. I feel like it is some sort of reunion! I am home just after lunch and have a good rest. The next morning I can hardly walk; I am in total agony and seriously question why I bothered having the injection at all. Matthew had said it would be very sore the next day and so I took some pain killers, rested as much as possible and low and behold the very next day, the pain had miraculously subsided.

It is amazing how quickly one's body recovers. I totally forget about my hip until several months later and even after the reconstructive surgery I am almost feeling normal. No, I can't feel certain parts of my stomach, but I have so much more movement in my right arm and much less tightness across the chest.

There was one slight disappointment. I had such a spare tyre of fat (well in fact I felt like I had a full set of sixteen articulated lorry tyres to be honest) that when I had my mobile phone on silent/vibrate mode, I could never feel it in my pocket and so very often used to miss phone calls. I was really hoping that once the fat was removed this problem would go away. However, this was not meant to be. Due to the numbness around the scar and the total lack of feeling in the stomach, I still cannot feel the phone vibrate and still miss lots of phone calls. So, if you have ever called me and I didn't answer, you now know why!

At the end of August, my brother and family from Lancashire come to stay and then we go off to Centre Parcs in the Netherlands with the Darnells. Just before we go I have my final check up with Adam Searle. He is very pleased with my progress and his handiwork. He can see that my new right breast is still higher than my newly reduced left one and he is a little unhappy with the shape of this, but tells me that he can tidy that up in phase two. He declares me fit and well to go on holiday and return to work. Excellent news.

Whilst we are away I limit my physical activities, but still manage to swim – a little – cycle and ski on a short indoor ski slope. Not bad at all, I feel. All the others (except Sarah) try snowboarding (I am definitely too old for that), waterskiing and wakeboarding. Now that I am definitely envious of – I have water-skied in the past, and would love to have done so again. However, there is no way my chest and stomach could have dealt with the holding on and being pulled along, let alone my hip when I would have fallen over.

There were only a few small mishaps on the holiday. Ed broke his wrist snowboarding; I fell onto my bike, landed on the wheel nut with my right leg which left a big dent in the muscle and Lizzie fell off her bike and ripped her knee open through two layers of denim! Apart from that, a fairly normal holiday.

CHAPTER 25

A Few Minor Adjustments Including the Dog Ears

The new academic year starts and I am training another teacher. I am working in year six again and love it: a whole new batch of children to get to know, enjoy and have fun with. Ron and I are working together again with a different support teacher, but now we just fall into the comfortable routine that we have got into. Truly he is the best partner I have worked with so far. Although I am back into the groove with work, I still feel I am marking time till I can finish getting my body back to normal.

At half term we go back to Dubai. Who can believe that it is two years since we were last here? I cannot believe that this time two years ago I was just getting ready to have the mastectomy. It is great to spend time with Stevi and Brian again; I do realise how much I miss my friend. I know she is just on the end of the phone, but it is just not the same.

We do all the touristy things, including going up the Burg Khalifa, the tallest building in the world and shopping at Dubai Mall, the biggest mall in the world. John, Stevi, Lizzie and Marcus have a go at indoor skydiving. You can do it in the UK, but it is so much cheaper in Dubai. I would have loved to go, but I am realising my sensible head has become much more sensible, or is it that my head is starting to listen to my body? Anyway, I don't have a go, I just photograph and film the others. It does look a lot of fun.

I have arranged an appointment with Adam Searle for the middle of November, having checked with my breast surgeon and oncologist before I did so, as I am due for my annual mammogram in January. They both feel it would be sensible to have the check before the next phase of surgery, as my chest will be too sore to be squeezed flat for several months after. The benefit of having a mastectomy is that I only need to have one breast checked now, as there is no mammary tissue in my new one, just stomach fat and that can't get breast cancer!

I go to see Adam about phase two of the rebuilding work, being all set check-up wise. John comes with me to see him and I have my little book in which I have written down all my questions ready. We have quite a long discussion about timing. He is of the opinion that if I wait a few more months then the new breast will gravitate southwards a little more. This would mean that he would be matching my left breast to something that was nearer to its final resting place. However, for me the timing of the surgery to minimise the inconvenience to school is at the front of my mind. Adam says kindly, that he will be happy to do it whenever I feel I want it done, with the understanding that it may not give the optimal final result.

We agree on early December. I want it as late as possible in the term; however, it needs to be when Adam and Kirsten will be around to manage the follow up, knowing that we will be falling into the Christmas period. This surgery we are going to have to pay for ourselves. Pru Health (the insurance company) only covers me for one reconstructive operation, even though it often takes two or three procedures, especially in larger breasted women. We decide this is something that we are prepared to pay for, as I might have to wait a very long time on the NHS and we can use some of the critical illness payout money for it.

Adam manages my expectation in terms of what he is going to

do. He will cut into the left breast through the scars he made last time and reduce the size a little more, to make the shape more symmetrical to my newly constructed right one. The nipple will be detached again and replaced in the optimal position. He will, using liposuction, adjust some unevenness in my tummy around the shark bite scar and also remove some of the fat from the 'dog ears', just above the scar line on both hips. Whilst he is there he will suck a little more fat out from my love handles and the middle section of my abdomen, above my new flat stomach and beneath my newly shaped pair of breasts. This will help to bring my figure back into proportion. The surgery should take two to three hours. I am booked in at the Lister Hospital in Chelsea for an overnight stay.

It is now the end of November and my hip is starting to hurt again. I am limping gently and John says I am starting to walk like my mother. She had been over seventy at the time; he does say the kindest things! Again I have to put this on the back burner until after I have had the breast surgery.

Operation day comes round quickly and John has the day off. We make our way by train to the hospital and I have the surgery at lunchtime. It is the same anaesthetist, David Chisholm, who put me to sleep back in the summer at the Royal Marsden. Adam comes up to see me with his magic marker and tape measure. As he draws he talks John and I through what he is actually going to do. I am taken down to theatre – a routine – with which I am way too familiar with now and chat away to David as he puts me to sleep. I tell him I am writing a book and he replies that he is also writing one. His is about Paediatric Anaesthesiology, something a little more erudite than mine. As we chat away, I drift off…

I wake up in recovery in much more pain than I am expecting, all over. I tell the nurses and they get me some tablets straight away. Later, when I am back in my room and David comes to see me, he tells me that because I cannot tolerate morphine, the type of drugs he has been using are much more difficult to calibrate. I am settling down now, so he is pleased.

I FELT A RIGHT ONE...

Adam comes to see me shortly after and shows me his handiwork. When I look down all I can see are two ginormous bruises on either side of my body. They are the size of basketballs. This is the result of the liposuction and it is this I notice before I actually look at my breast. The fact that I am wearing a support bra which has elastic that goes down to my belly button is fascinating. Not too sexy, but then what would you expect for hospital attire? I have one drain in on the left breast, but Adam tells me it will come out tomorrow before I go home. He feels it is unlikely to drain too much and it turns out that he is right.

John goes home not long before I have my dinner. I watch some TV and update my friends of my progress on Facebook. Although I had joined Facebook over a year ago, as the only way I was going to let my thirteen year old daughter onto it was if I was her friend, I had not actually spent too much time on it. This had changed during the last few months and when I am sitting at the PC doing my lesson planning for school, I normally have Facebook on in the background. It has been brilliant recently as I have reconnected with a whole host of friends from primary school who live all over the world. Rowena, my friend who now lives in California, had posted some photos of us having a sleepover when I was about ten which I had never seen. I then scanned in the photos I had taken when I left Heathfield, my primary school, in 1972. We ended up having a massively long conversation between us all across three continents. Now that is what Facebook is for. Anyway, when you're sitting on your own in a hospital room, it is a great way to keep yourself happy.

On Wednesday morning, John drives up to London, picks me up and brings me home. I am quite sore, but nothing a few pain killers won't knock on the head. At least the pain in my body takes my mind off the pain in my hip!

By Friday I am starting to react to the plaster they have used to cover over the nipple and keep it attached, so I arrange to go up and see Kirsten to redress the wounds. The following week I go back to see Adam for a check-up and have some of the stitches out. I also go into school a couple of times to see the children before Christmas and give them the presents I had got them consisting of pens and note pads.

Then it is the Christmas holidays. The day after term finishes is the day that all the snow comes down. It is freezing; minus nine degrees and huge quantities of snow. John and I get stuck in Waitrose car park in South Harrow, but luckily we have snow socks for our front tyres in the boot of the car. *Why*? I hear you ask. Well, they are left over from last year's skiing holiday and they had never been taken out of the car, lucky us! We get them out and hey presto, they work like magic. Even though it takes us over an hour and a half to get back from shopping, we at least do it without skidding all over the place. I have never had so many people point at me (well not me, but the car) and give me covetous looks in all my life.

I have one more visit to have stitches out before Christmas and then it is getting all the final bits ready before heading to Lancashire to stay with the Motes of the north for the holidays. All is well until the 23rd, when I get the twenty-four hour vomiting bug that is doing the rounds. Sarah kindly cooks John and the children dinner and on the way home at about 10pm, John falls over on the sheet ice that is still lying on all the roads and pavements away from the main roads.

I am, by now, sitting downstairs in my jim jams watching TV, when Marcus rushes in and says, "I think Dad has broken his leg."

An ashen faced John is half carried in by Ed and Sarah and sits heavily down on the sofa. I gently ease his sock off, take one look at his leg and say "That's broken, I'd better get dressed and take you to hospital".

John looks at me and winces. Marcus gets him some pain killers and we put an ice pack on it quickly. I am still very sore and there is no way I will be able to get John out of the car on my own when we get to the hospital, so we depart for a visit to Northwick Park A&E for a family outing!

I FELT A RIGHT ONE...

We are there by 10.30 and John gets triaged and sent for an x-ray in less than an hour. A & E is really busy and there is an estimated three hour wait. By about 2.00am on Christmas Eve, John gets called through and the doctor tells him that yes, he has broken the bottom of the fibula, the smaller of the two bones in the ankle. We wait a little while longer for a nurse to plaster it and then we make it home at about 3.15am. Wow, what a day.

We have a good lie in the next morning. John calls work and lets them know that he won't be in the following week until he goes back to the fracture clinic. They are so busy, in fact I saw three people leave casualty with plasters on arms and legs before John, so it is no wonder that there are no appointments until after New Year.

The children pack the car up for us and we drive up to our friends in Tring for our annual Christmas Eve social event. We go early so John can get a seat. He gets lots of sympathy, laced with a little bit of laughter and has everyone waiting on him hand and foot, well, mostly foot!

We leave the Warren household at about 6.30pm and go cross country from Tring to meet the A40 at Bicester. Then it is a straightforward drive up the M40, M42, M6 to Junction 28 where we get off for Leyland. The roads are really clear and we do it in about three hours. When we get to Justin's house, it is minus ten degrees. The snow is so powdery they have not even been able to make a snow man because the snow is too dry! It doesn't seem as icy as Harrow, maybe because it hasn't got above zero since it snowed and so has not melted into ice.

Luckily, Justin and Jo's spare room is downstairs and there is a loo too, which means that John only has to go upstairs when he wants a bath. He has to bath, which he hates, because he cannot risk getting his plaster wet. We have a fantastic Christmas with the Motes and they spoil both John and I rotten. I am totally shattered on Christmas Day after the long drive and very sore all over. My two children love spending time with their cousins and when the Motes return from church we have general present opening time.

A Few Minor Adjustments Including the Dog Ears

We would normally go for lovely long walks whilst we stay in Lancashire, but with John's foot and my hip, we aren't going anywhere in a hurry. I do manage to drag the children round the park on Boxing Day, whilst Justin and Jo go further afield for a more extended walk.

Too soon it is time to return home and we hit the road at about 11.00am on the Bank Holiday Monday. All I can say is that it is the journey from hell. It takes six and a half hours. I had planned to do some food shopping when we get home, needless to say it will have to wait till tomorrow.

The next day we are due to go for a walk in Richmond Park with friends. We are meeting in the Pembroke Lodge car park. Jane and Tony know about John's broken leg but it comes as a total surprise to Paul, who bursts into uncontrollable laughter at John's misfortune. The irony of coming for a walk on crutches has us all in stitches. Lizzie stays to keep John company with a cup of coffee whilst Marcus and I join the walk. It is only now that I realise how bad my hip really is. I am limping more and more noticeably and the stabbing pains, if I catch my leg in the wrong position, are excruciating. We really don't walk that far, but it is more than enough for me and I lag behind everyone else. I am sure if I wasn't there they would have walked considerably further.

Tony and I walk slowly back to the Lodge to get John and Lizzie and then drive to the Roebuck Pub at the top of Richmond Hill for a lovely lunch. It is a dog friendly pub and the pooches sit quietly under the table, waiting patiently, whilst we all tuck into some scrummy food.

On New Year's Eve, I go to see Kirsten to get the last of my stitches out. She is happy with the progress of my wounds and I am now fine until I see Adam for a check up in the middle of February. We have a relaxing weekend after having Eamonn, Zoe and the children and the Spalding family over for New Years Eve, then first thing on Tuesday 4th I take John back to the fracture clinic.

It is by far the busiest clinic I think I have ever seen in a hospital and there is standing room only. We get seen relatively quickly and sent for a new x-ray. When we get back from that, it is time for a new plaster to be put on – this time of fibre glass and then we have a discussion with the doctor. He explains everything clearly and it seems to me that John is lucky not to have to have an operation. The large triangle of bone that had broken off the bottom of the fibula is noticeably separated from the rest of the bone.

On crutches and still non weight-bearing for another three weeks will mean John cannot be completely mobile till the end of January – nearly five weeks after the actual break. The thing that annoys me the most is that there are at least three people on crutches having to stand up. I want to shout across the clinic that if you are a visitor with a patient then you should stand up and give your seat to one of the three people who obviously have broken legs and who are left standing. Incredible!

With John being the invalid now, I help him and I feel glad that I am able to give back to him just a small amount of the support that he has given me over the last couple of years.

In the second week of January, John and I go to a fiftieth birthday party of a friend who normally lives in Australia. We seem to be going to a lot of these now. In fact I will be having my very own later this year! It is a great evening and I see some people who I have not seen for over thirty years. It seems really naughty to go out on a school night, but for such a special occasion it is more than worth how tired you feel the next day. The only problem for me is the standing; I actually don't sit down all evening and by the time we get home, my hip and knees hurt so much I can hardly walk. I determine that I will call Matthew Bartlett's secretary tomorrow and get her to ask him to refer me to a hip specialist. This just cannot go on.

I get my referral and make the first available appointment, which is next Thursday. The pain is so bad now that I am walking with a pronounced limp and if I have been sitting down for a while then it takes me some time to straighten up and limp away. The pain is really starting to get me down, it is almost as bad as when I had shingles during chemo, but at least if I don't move the pain is much less. Unfortunately, being a teacher I actually move quite a lot. I try to sit down as much as possible at school. I get the children to do more and even start asking other people to carry things for me. This feels so alien to me as I have always been strong and capable. Even when I had cancer it did not feel so debilitating as having this constant background and then moments of searing pain.

The following week, John starts to go back into work for four hours a day. He goes in and back by taxi to Slough. I can see he is pleased to be able to be back at work, even though it seems to me that he is doing just as much at home. However, as he is home by mid afternoon, he comes with me to see the hip consultant, Simon Jennings.

As it turns out, it is the same consultant John is under at Northwick Park only he hasn't got to see him, but has seen his registrar. I am by now in so much pain that walking is as painful to watch me do as it is to actually do. John is at least four times faster than me with his crutches!

Simon sits us down, looks at the scan that I had done last May with Matthew Bartlett and reads through the radiologist's report. He does a physical examination as well, through which I wince and whimper. He discusses the options bluntly, but would like me to have more tests before he makes a final recommendation. He basically describes me as crippled, which I am, but I guess I just don't want to admit it. He talks about two options: an arthroscopy to go in and tidy things up, which he feels would have limited benefit, or a hip replacement.

A hip replacement! At forty-nine. A hip replacement. I am shocked. I know I shouldn't be, as Matthew Bartlett had also mentioned it last year. I guess I am just not ready to take it in. Tears start to trickle down my cheeks. He comments that he knows this is difficult for me to hear, especially after everything I have been through in the last two years, but it is a serious consideration.

I FELT A RIGHT ONE...

He gives me the paperwork to get an x-ray, CT scan and another MRI of my hip and also says I need another cortisone injection to help with the pain. I ask if I have to have a general anaesthetic for this, but he says I can have one done with a local, which is a great relief. He says he will see me when I have the results of the tests. We walk off to the Imaging Department to organise the tests.

I am devastated. I don't know why, but I am a teary wreck for the rest of the evening and feel incredibly low. I actually feel worse than I did when I was told I had cancer, if you can believe it. I am sure that some of it is the weariness of the constant and not insignificant pain that I am in. It is tiring and just gets to you; it also affects my sleep, which due to hot flushes and the regular need for the loo is not good at the best of times. I am just really tired and I definitely have a feeling of *it is not fair, why me? Haven't I gone through enough?* As I am thinking this, I hate that I feel this way. It really is not like me and I am cross and frustrated with myself, which makes me feel even more miserable.

Tearily, I ask John, "if this is what I am like when I am forty-nine, what will I be like when I am sixty-five?"

"Bionic!" he replies swiftly with a smile. I give him a weak and wobbly grin in return.

When I get home I phone Zoe and Anne. Zoe is a medical secretary for a highly renowned knee surgeon. I wanted her opinion and for her to ask her boss what he thinks of the consultant I am seeing. I phone Anne because she has been a medical secretary for her whole life and has worked with Orthopaedic guys for many years. Anne is pragmatic and thinks I should also speak to my oncologist. I know she is worried in case there is anything underlying my symptoms that is not just arthritis related.

The next day when I go into school, my head is still not in the right place. I go to tell Chris and Gill. They must be totally sick of hearing about my ailments and what is going wrong with my body. I burst into tears when I tell Chris; it just shows how fed up I really am. I know the 'feeling down' won't last long and I will bounce back, I always do, but I don't like feeling low. It just doesn't suit me. I don't even have the energy to feel angry. I need to get my head around how I feel and how I am going to deal with this. It is not so much the having a serious hip condition, as the bloody inconvenience of it all.

During a lesson I am teaching this Friday morning, I realise something. I have been teaching the children in PSHE (Personal, Social and Health Education) about a theory I came across many years ago whilst working in commerce; the doughnut theory, as I like to call it, but I think it is called the 'circle of influence and the circle of concern.' It reminds me that I need to be more proactive with how I deal with the issues that are affecting me, rather than reactive.

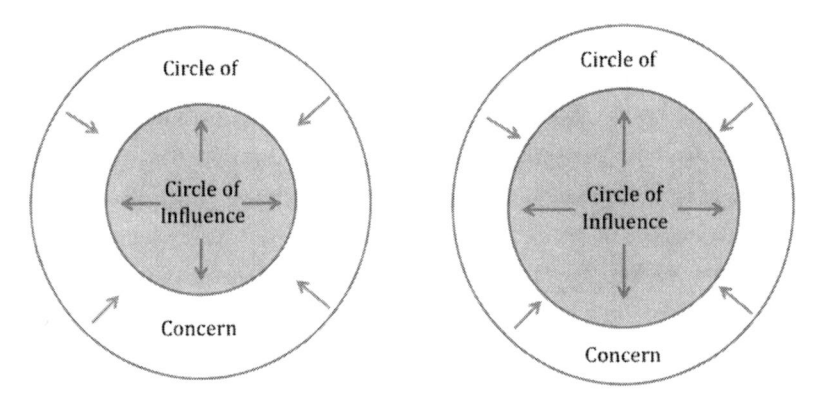

The bigger the ring of the doughnut, the more stress you feel, the smaller the thickness of the ring, the less stress you feel.

Figure 1: The Doughnut

Basically, the theory is that anxiety and worry are like a doughnut. If you are concerned about something then you need either to be proactive by increasing the amount of influence you have over the issue, or reduce the amount you are worrying about it. The objective

I FELT A RIGHT ONE...

is to make the ring of the doughnut as thin or non-existent as possible. The view is that by being proactive you can increase the amount of influence you have over things and therefore have a positive impact. The opposite is also true, that if you are reactive then the doughnut can get bigger, which means an increase in stress. Of course, it is a bit difficult for me to actually regenerate cartilage and bone, so I guess I had better stop worrying about it and just get it sorted. The sooner I get it sorted, the sooner the doughnut will disappear and, most importantly, the pain.

Sorry, lesson over, back to the current situation.

I do over the weekend email my oncologist's secretary, just to update him. That little niggle in the back of your mind – is this something more sinister? – just starts to creep in. I think back to what Michael Burke said about when you have persistent problems and how it might make you feel. He was right; your mind plays tricks on you, even though you try to control it. The rational part of your brain knows you are potentially overreacting, but the emotional part cannot help itself. Perhaps my mind goes in that direction because I need a reason for why my hip has deteriorated so badly in the last couple of years.

This weekend we treat ourselves to going to the cinema without the children. I can honestly say, I have not watched a film without a single child in the audience for so long I cannot remember. What a pleasure! We go to see *The King's Speech* and thoroughly enjoy ourselves. Afterwards John and I walk, if you can call it that, to Starbucks for a coffee and a light lunch. By now, walking is incredibly difficult and terribly slow. The fact that John can go four times as fast as me on crutches makes us both giggle. Surely anyone looking at the pair of us must wonder what on earth has happened, we must look like we have been in a car crash or some other major disaster and they must be trying to work out who has come off worse!

CHAPTER 26

No You Don't Have Bone Cancer, You Just Need a Hip Replacement

On Monday afternoon, I go for all the scans and most importantly for the pain killing cortisone injection, which this time is being done under a local anaesthetic. It is painful, even with the pain relief, but it is fascinating as I get to watch it happening, on the x-ray screen, as it is being done. I have almost immediate relief from the pain; I am sure it is the local anaesthetic, but it is wonderful. I walk out with a considerably smaller limp. Yippee! When I get home there is an email from my oncologist asking me to go for an appointment tomorrow.

As I am very sore after the local anaesthetic wears off I actually don't go into school the next day. I rest my hip so that the injection can work its magic and help the pain. John's mum takes him to the fracture clinic and he comes home with an air cast on, which he is delighted about. He is home in under an hour which is amazingly good for Northwick Park.

In the afternoon, we go up to the hospital together to see Nihal Shah, my oncologist. Of course, I know why he wants to see me.

I FELT A RIGHT ONE...

He wants to make sure that what is going on with my hip is not metastatic bone cancer. He is very thorough, asks lots of questions and says he wants me to have a full work-up of tests – Blood, bone scan and body CT. He is fairly confident that it is not cancer, but needs me to have all the tests in order to rule it out completely. I had not really thought of this myself until the weekend, when I had sent him the email. I know I should have considered the possibility sooner, but because I mostly see the positive in things, I guess I just don't let my mind wander into the negatives places to where it can so easily go.

Again I go to the imaging department to arrange the appointments. I reckon I am going for the world record number of different tests one can have in a week. The bone scan is arranged for Thursday and the CT scan for Saturday.

On Thursday I have to go to the hospital at midday for the radioactive injection back to school to teach for a while (and drink a litre of water) and then return to the hospital at three for the scan. It is the lovely physicist who did my sentinel node biopsy; I remember him and he remembers me. All in all it takes about half an hour or so and I am back at school by 4.00pm.

On Saturday I go for my CT scan at 10.30, only to be sent away to come back in a couple of hours as I had totally forgotten to fast and had eaten a bowl of muesli for breakfast this morning. What a moron! I do giggle when the receptionist greeted me by name without even looking at the screen or my file. It just shows you how many times I have been to that department in the last couple of years.

I go back at 12.30 and find that this is an interesting test, as I have to drink about half a litre of special liquid which after about 15 minutes coats all the key organs in my body that they need to check, particularly the liver and kidneys. I then am taken into the CT scanning room, for the second time in a week! For this test I need an injection of Iodine (like I had before my reconstruction last year). The radiographer tries to find a vein, but it is freezing in the room (where is a hot flush when you really need one?) and even though she has covered me with a blanket my veins just do not want to play ball. Nothing doing at the elbow she tries the wrist gets the needle in, but it doesn't work.

She goes off and gets a doctor. He has two attempts and finally gets the needle in to the back of my hand. I am in tears by the end; they are very apologetic, but it is not their fault I have crap veins and they can't use the lovely juicy ones in my right arm! I am going to look like a pin cushion. The radiographer reminds me that when the iodine goes it will make me feel like I desperately want to go to the loo. It does.

When I am finished, my left arm looks like I have been shooting up drugs and is going to produce some excellent bruises.

On Tuesday I go back to see Nihal Shah. Lizzie comes in with me as I have to take her to the orthodontist straight afterwards. He smiles when he tells me that all the tests have come back totally clear, except for the fact that I obviously have significant degeneration of the right hip joint, which is osteoarthritic. This I already know.

It is really great to know that I am still cancer free. I knew I was, but having all the tests does put your mind on edge and make you think about things you don't really want to think about. The really positive impact that having all these tests has created is that now I feel like a hip replacement is not the end of the world, which is completely different to how I felt two weeks ago. It has eliminated that small, tiny little nag that sits in the back of your mind – *is it cancer? What will I do if it is? Not it can't be, don't be so silly.* This potential problem allows me to put things back into perspective. It really could have been so much worse, it is only a hip replacement that I can now handle.

I don't have to see Nihal now for a year and my breast surgeon for six months. So, again, every cloud has a silver lining. I have had a full cancer MOT, is what I like to think. This is great news. Now I know I am ready to deal with whatever Simon Jennings feels I need to have done. If it is a hip replacement, then so be it.

I FELT A RIGHT ONE...

On Thursday afternoon John and I go back to see Simon Jennings. He can immediately see that I am walking better and asks how much the cortisone has helped. He shows us all the scans and talks through what the radiographer's report says. He thinks that I might have had some damage before I had chemo, but that the chemo itself may have been the cause of the accelerated decline. Whatever the cause, we still have to decide what to do. The problem is that I have cysts in the bone of the hip itself, plus loss of cartilage to the inside of the joint and the head of the femur (thigh bone). He could do an arthroscopy and tidy up the cartilage but this would not solve the bone cyst problem, has nearly as long a recovery time as a hip replacement and most importantly he cannot guarantee would be much help. He would recommend the full replacement.

We discuss how much recuperation is needed and the impacts on what I can and cannot do in the future. It won't stop me swimming (except breast stroke, which I am not allowed to do anyway, because of my bad lower back) cycling, or skiing. In fact it will within two to three months mean that I am pain free. The obvious question is how long will it last? He would like to give me a metal joint which is coated in a ceramic compound and this should last longer than I do. Excellent, I hope I last a very long time.

I ask how many cortisone injections you can have. This, he says, is a good question, because managing the pain is going to be the thing that determines when I have the operation.

The question is when should I have it done? There is never a good time to take six to eight weeks out of work, is there? At the moment I am driving the 600 metres to school, because even after the cortisone, I am still in some pain and definitely still limping because of it. The pain relief had worked really well for the first week, but for some reason after sitting on a stool in the computer suite at school for teacher training, when I got up, the hip was agony and has not been so good since. In fact after sitting at the swimming pool for an hour and a half on Wednesday, I could barely walk again. The sooner I get it done, the better.

Who would have thought that I would be happy to hear I need a hip replacement? Certainly not me. It could have been much worse and I know I am lucky. My cancer has not come back and it is just plain bad luck that I need to have more major surgery less than a year after the last. Four in two and a half years is not bad going.

It is interesting though. This whole episode has made me analyse different significant health issues. On the one hand you have cancer – a horrible disease which messes with your mind and certainly requires pretty disgusting treatment, but does not involve much pain in the grand scheme of things. On the other hand you have a major joint problem, which is a nightmare as it does not just affect walking but bending, turning, sleeping. It is painful, very painful and constant pain is debilitating. I can honestly say that apart from the psychological impact that breast cancer gave me, the physical part was not nearly as bad as this (apart from the bout of shingles). At the moment I am a cripple. I am the heaviest I have ever been and the most unfit I have been since I can remember. I hate it. I am not saying I want cancer again, of course not. I am just saying that each illness has its down sides and I must say I think constant pain is harder to deal with than anything else. You only realise how pain affects you when it goes, or is taken away. The cortisone does this for me, it makes me realise what I have been letting myself put up with for some time. Sometimes when the pain creeps up on you, like it has done with me, you don't notice how bad it has become until you can barely walk.

John, of course, says he is not at all surprised by what Simon Jennings said. "Remember," he says "I can see you walk, you can't."

I say to him, "So after 'Cancer Scabby Face' and 'Cancer Booby Chest', what are you going to call me now, 'Cripple Gammy Hip?'" We both laugh out loud.

The next morning I go into school and find Gill and Chris to have a conversation. The plan is to wait until after SATs, which means the end of May.

I FELT A RIGHT ONE...

By now I am in full swing organising a dinner dance to raise money for the hospice. I have organised musicians and a DJ who have all donated their time for nothing. Raffle and auction prizes have also been generously donated by many friends. The only issue is getting people to buy the tickets. The price is set at £35 per head, which includes a welcome drink and soft drinks on the table. My trustee colleague at St Luke's, Ash, helped me find the venue. A surprising place in the middle of Wealdstone, called Premier Banqueting, which is used for Asian weddings. It is beautiful and I know that when everyone actually gets there they will think that it is good value for money. However, you can actually see the recession biting now; £35 is a lot of money for an evening out for so many people.

Just before half term I go back to visit Adam Searle for my six week post surgery check up. He sees me limp in and asks what the problem is. When I tell him about my hip, I can see him thinking and I already know what is going through his head. "Don't worry," I say, "the best words my oncologist could give me were 'The good news is you don't have bone cancer, but your orthopaedic surgeon is right, it looks like a hip replacement might be in order'."

He sighs and smiles and tells me he had been working out how to ask me if I had got myself checked out, as his first thought had been what the cause of the problem was. The discussion of when I will get my nipple rebuilt seems much less important now. Adam is really happy with the shape of the left breast now and I must admit, so am I. He chats about how my new right one is still higher than he would like, but is confident that it will drop over time. He even tells me about how in the past he and his team had felt they were reconstructing breasts that were a little too low. Now he is wondering if they have overcooked it a little and perhaps he is making them a little too high. He says he will need to have a discussion with his team about what they will need to do in the future.

It must be so hard; each woman must be different, depending

on her age and the strength and elasticity of tissue. I think he has done a brilliant job and so what if they are just a little uneven? After all, I don't walk around naked do I? Just as well really, as it would not be a pretty sight. When I wear a bra it is hardly noticeable. An additional benefit of not having such a large chest that I have not realised until now is that people, by that I mostly men mostly, do not stare at that area of my body quite so much. Mind you, would men really notice that they were slightly different in size anyway? Sorry, that is sexist and mean! Another great benefit of a smaller chest is the effect it has had on my back. I get so much less back pain and discomfort. I totally understand why so many women with large chests would choose to have reductions, in order to improve their posture and back comfort.

Adam explains to me how he will rebuild the nipple by taking a small circle of skin, lifting it up, then taking out a narrow strip of skin from each side of the circle that has been removed. These are left attached right by the nipple, but twisted and curved round the edge of the circle of skin that has been lifted up. The ends are joined together and then the circle of skin placed on top, all the joins stitched neatly and finally, the two gaps at either side are then pulled tight together, just leaving two small scars which will be covered by the tattoo of the areola. In my mind, all I can see is the circle and a slits either side. I comment that to me, it will look much like a London tube logo.

He smiles at me and says laughingly, "Now I am never going to be able to think about this type of nipple reconstruction without thinking of a tube sign ever again!"

We agree to leave the nipple for the moment, as getting my hip sorted is the priority. It will also give my new right breast longer to settle down anyway.

In the build up to the dinner dance, I need to buy a new evening dress. In fact, I have been feeling a lot better about my body now and truly believe I have a better figure than when I started all this. Yes, I still carry more weight than I would like, but I am really delighted with the fact that I have a flat stomach and a noticeable waist now. I go shopping with Lizzie and a friend to a local boutique, where I have always been able to find something when all else fails. You tell the ladies what you are looking for and they find something to meet your needs. I start with a gorgeous red dress with a tight bodice covered in sequins, it is lovely. I then proceed to try on a selection of half a dozen other outfits, but end up with the first one. I am delighted and can honestly say that I could never have worn this dress before I had my reconstructive surgery. I need to go braless and I can. It again makes me realise how much physical benefit I have gained from the whole process; I really do have a better figure and this dress just goes to show it.

My poor friends, colleagues and neighbours must be so fed up of me nagging them to buy tickets, but slowly the sales start to increase and many, many people who are unable or don't want to come, start donating. The only problem is that we have promised the venue 300 people. Bless them, they are happy with the 160 people we drum up and we just compromise on some of the extras they were going to include. I also pull in every favour I can for raffle tickets, auction prizes and my friends really come up with the goods.

A couple of weeks before the dinner dance my hip is really starting to get sore again. I email my surgeon's secretary and she arranges for me to have the paperwork to get another cortisone injection the following week. This is the last one I can have. The Wednesday before the dinner I have the injection. It does not help nearly as much this time – a slight improvement in the pain, but not much. I ask my surgeon what type of pain killers I can take that are stronger.

Finally, the day has arrived and from 3.00pm we are able to access the venue to complete the final set up, including the band and DJ. One of the funniest things that happens during the evening is when we play a game called 'heads or tails'. This is where anyone who wants to play pays a pound, then a coin is tossed and you put your hands on your head if you think it will come up heads or your hands on your bottom if you think it will come up tails. If you are wrong you sit down and then you play the next round until the final person standing wins and gets the prize of a bottle of champagne.

I get Hunty to run this game as he, I know, has done it lots of times before and it is a break for people from hearing my voice all the time. During the game, Hunty reminds people that we are having this to raise money. He comments that the last time he had seen me with a microphone was twenty years ago at a ball he had organised. I had received a cheque from someone and put it down my cleavage. It had disappeared, never to be seen again. I quickly grab the microphone from him and respond with, "Do you know what he did the day after I had my mastectomy? He sent me a text message saying, 'Has the cheque turned up yet?'"

Everybody roars with laughter and then I realise what I have just said to everyone. Obviously most people in the room know about my personal circumstances, but now I have just told everyone else. I hadn't thought, but do you know, I don't really care. The story was true, funny and just seemed the right thing to say at the time. Anyway Hunty started it and I had to finish it.

Heads and tails is complete and everyone goes to the buffet for their main course. There is a choice of Indian, Chinese and English cuisine. The curry is the most popular and it is delicious. I find myself being the maitre d'hôtel and organising the order that the tables go up in. It is a lovely chance to catch up with people I have not had a chance to meet and thank for coming. I know the majority personally, except the guests of friends and a few brave people who had bought tickets from the St Luke's website.

After the main course, we promote a couple of other fundraising activities and the children go round promoting the raffle tickets. I act as the auctioneer for the five key auction lots and then ask a range of people to draw out raffle tickets. It is then time for the band to come on and finally I can relax. I realise I have not actually had an alcoholic drink yet as I had not wanted to risk not being sharp, but now I feel I can indulge in just one. I will be driving home so that will be my limit. The guests have made a huge effort and we have a wide range of multi-cultural outfits, which really adds to the visual effect for the evening. It all winds up at midnight and the band and the disco take an hour or so to pack up. I leave in my car and unload all the things at home, then fall into bed.

The next morning I count all the money and all in all we have raised £5,087 in total. I am delighted, but I know that this is an event that you can only organise every few years as pulling in the level of favour I did for this is not something that you can do very often.

Adrenaline is a wonderful thing and I reckon it kept the pain in my hip away, however, as soon as the dinner dance is over the pain comes back with a vengeance. The injection does not really seem to have had much effect at all this time. I call my surgeon's secretary and ask if it is possible to bring the operation forward at all. I was scheduled for the end of May and she is able to bring it forward by a month, so I am booked in for the end of April – the day before the royal wedding and the long weekend.

Before then we have a short holiday booked. John and I are going away with some friends to Marrakech for a long weekend before Easter. It is the first time we have had a holiday of any sort without our children. We had been away overnight about once a year since they were born, but this was for three nights. They were going to stay with Sarah, round the corner. I am worried about all the walking with my hip, so the surgeon kindly prescribes some significantly stronger painkillers to keep me going until the surgery. It is only three weeks away now.

The purpose of this short break is to celebrate three fiftieth birthdays, one of which is mine. The trip has been planned since last October and I am glad that I can still go. So, in the middle of April we head off. It is a fantastic weekend and we stay in an old Riyadh in the middle of the Medina (the old city). Jane and Anita have done most of the organising and have done a fantastic job. It is the first time that we have been away on holiday with this group of friends. We have been away with Jane and Tony to play golf before, but not with the others. It is a fantastic weekend and spending time with such old friends is really special. We spend a lot of time discussing friendship and the value and benefit that it has in our lives. It makes me realise how truly lucky I am; friends are so important to me and over the last couple of years they have proven invaluable. I have garnered strength, almost osmosis-like, from my friends without even realising it. The warmth and generosity of spirit that they have provided me with has been like an invisible blanket of comfort that I am still feeling the benefit of.

My friends seem to think that I have been brave and dealt with cancer, and all the issues that it brings, in an admirable way. Yet, to me, I have just gotten on with life as normally as possible. What else could I do? Give up, mope, moan, scream, rant and complain that life is not fair? Well life is not fair and so many people have so many issues to deal with. Training to be a teacher has taught me this. Children have so much to cope with nowadays. I am no longer surprised by some of the home situations that they have to deal with and to me they are handling things that have way more serious implications than having cancer has.

This holiday really makes me reflect that living life to the full is so important. I want to make sure that I really do live life to the fullest that I can. Take every opportunity to do things now, not wait. As the saying goes, why put off till tomorrow what you can do today? It is so right.

CHAPTER 27

We Can Rebuild You Phase II

In no time at all the holiday is over, I go back to school and make sure that everything is sorted for the children before they take their SATs tests. I then finish on Wednesday and go into hospital on Thursday morning. I am due in at lunchtime, but we have time to stop of at the mobility shop in Harrow to buy some essential items for post surgery. We need to buy chair and bed raisers, a solid cushion, a toilet seat raiser, a picker-up thing and a device to help put socks on! As I am having a hip replacement they are allowed to sell it all to me without VAT. Whilst we are at the shop, we bump into a neighbour who has already had the same surgery and when she finds out what I am doing she is very encouraging. It is actually sinking in now that I am about to have another major operation. I know it is going to help, but the process of getting there is not something I am looking forward to.

I am due to have the surgery late in the afternoon. John takes me up and we go through the all too familiar booking in process. The anaesthetist comes to see me and when my pulse and blood pressure are checked my pressure is a little high. Not surprising really – I am sure I suffer from white coat syndrome, the minute that someone in a medical uniform comes near me my blood pressure shoots through the roof!

The surgeon comes to see me and I sign all the consent forms and remind him that he needs to take some photos. I had asked if I could keep the top of the femur when they cut it off, but the hospital policy is that it is clinical waste and I cannot keep it. I had wanted to have it made into a paper weight as a reminder of how amazing medical science actually is, but it is not to be.

I go down to surgery and I don't even remember coming back through recovery. I wake up and John is in the room smiling at me. I am definitely in pain and I take a quick look down at my leg. The bruising is substantial and it is also really swollen, but what had I expected. Simon comes to check that I am OK and tells me he is really happy with how the operation went and smiled when he told me he had some photos. He confirmed that the head of the femur was really bad and definitely would have been the cause of all my pain.

I have to use the bed pan that night, but the next morning the physio arrives to help me get out of bed. John is there already and comments, "Blimey, I break my ankle and am not allowed to weight bear for at least six weeks, but they cut the top of your femur off and you are supposed to walk the next day!"

I smile and inch my way over to the edge of the bed, ready to try to do what the physio tells me. She has a zimmer frame ready so I put my feet into my slippers and stand up. I take a few uncomfortable steps and then the world starts to spin. John and the physio grab my arms and manage to get me back to the bed before I nearly pass out. I feel really sick and wibbly-wobbly. The physio tells me not to worry and that we can try again tomorrow. The annoying thing is that I will have to use a bed pan, I hate them.

The next day I try again to walk, but still can only manage a few steps before I feel sick and faint. The nurses call my surgeon and they test my blood. Apparently, the younger you are the more blood you lose when having a hip replacement and it turns out I need a blood transfusion. Later on that afternoon I am given two units of blood and almost immediately I feel better. When the physio arrives the next morning, I am raring to go. I manage to walk round the corner to the physiotherapy room and even manage the small set of stairs in there. I am so happy that I almost do a dance.

Staying in hospital this time goes more slowly. I have fewer visitors; only, I am sure, because it is a long bank holiday weekend. I also think the time has dragged because I have been so immobile and feeling crap. Again, it is the nurses who make the time bearable. I get talking to one of the night nurses, who it turns out has also had breast cancer. She had told almost no-one. It must be hard getting sick when you are in the medical profession and working with people who know exactly what might be wrong with you. We talk for hours and I find her inspirational. Chloe (who nursed me during my mastectomy operation) and Elaine Sasto, the breast care nurse, also come to visit me, which is really sweet.

Simon, is happy for me to be discharged on Tuesday and I cannot wait. The swelling is starting to go down now and I am walking with crutches and have also tried with walking sticks. I feel I am limping, as if my new hip has made my right leg longer. I have to work really hard at not limping. It's going to take a while. John collects me on Tuesday morning and works from home that day. He has put all the leg raisers on the chairs as well as on the bed and bought another toilet seat so that I can use either the upstairs or downstairs loo. The strangest thing is sleeping on the other side of the bed. I have to sleep on the side I have had the replacement on for at least six weeks. It will make it easier for me to get in and out of bed.

It is important to keep moving and make sure that I do all the exercises I have been given. I cannot bend my hip joint more than ninety degrees for six weeks and I cannot take my knee across the midline of my body. This is to make sure that I don't dislocate my hip until all the scar tissue has formed, which will protect against this. Until you can't move in this way, it is impossible to realise how often you do these things naturally. I actually cannot put a sock on my right foot without the gadget and trying to sit comfortably is quite difficult, however as the days pass everything gets easier. The acute pain wears off and slowly I start doing more.

I go into school to start writing my reports and working on end of term projects. At four weeks post operation I am allowed to drive again and just six weeks after the surgery I am back at work in class. The way I look at it, I was in more pain prior to the surgery than I am now so why not? I start physiotherapy too. The main crippling pain has gone, but I am still suffering from a very specific pain in one of my hip flexor tendons. I am really keen to get this sorted as we are due to fly to Australia at the end of July.

After I got cancer, when we got some life insurance money I had said to John that we should do something special. I wanted to do some things that I had always dreamed of doing; things on my bucket list, if you like. Back in February, when I knew I was going to have the surgery in May, we had planned a trip to Australia for a month in August. John would only be able to come for three weeks, but it would be the trip of a lifetime and something that the children would remember forever.

Four weeks after surgery, John and the children drive up to London with me. I have been selected for interview as a volunteer for the London 2012 Olympics. I had applied last year immediately when you were allowed. I had had to change my original interview because it would only have been two weeks after surgery, but I felt now that with walking sticks I could manage. The whole process is impressively organised and I find myself being interviewed by a delightful man who works in IT and is a governor at a primary school in Hillingdon. The questions are aimed at assessing your suitability for being a volunteer in general and then one specifically for the area of expertise I am being interviewed for: press operations.

One of the questions he asks me is how I have dealt with adversity and I ask him if undertaking a mini-triathlon five days into radiotherapy counted. You see, I can use having cancer to my advantage! I really enjoy the process and he kindly ends by assuring me that if I am not selected to be a volunteer then he can't think who would be. I am really pleased.

Back at work, although I am really pleased with how much

the pain has been relieved and I can walk unaided without a limp, I am still suffering more pain than I had expected and am a little disappointed, to be honest. What can I do? I have just got to get on with life. The most important thing for me is to make sure that I will be fit enough to learn to scuba dive. Whilst I was at home after surgery, I had spent time sorting out the details of the trip. I now needed to sort out my medical so that I could actually dive. The dive company had given me the details of a doctor in Cairns. I had emailed her and asked about what her concerns were. Basically, having had radiotherapy, there is a risk of a specific lung condition. She seemed to think that having already survived breast cancer; I should not take any more risks with my health. She just does not get it; the whole point now is to live life to the full as much as I can and learning to dive is something I have wanted to do since I was a child. Jacques Cousteau has a lot to answer for.

At the end of June I go to my god daughter Kitty's eighteenth birthday party and I catch up with an old friend who I know is a very proficient scuba diver. I ask his advice and he gives me the email address of a doctor in London, who specialises in medicals for diving, and who he has used many times.

When I get home I email him immediately. Within a couple of days I hear back and arrange an appointment at the Hospital of St John and Elizabeth in St John's Wood. Within the hospital is a department called The London Dive Chamber. The doctor is brilliant; he sees it as his job to make sure that he certifies, as many people as possible as fit. He checks my ears and lungs. The likelihood of my having micro pulmonary fibrosis, which is what you can get from having radiotherapy, is very small and he passes me to dive. He says my restricted movement and loss in leg strength should not be an issue if I tell the dive school.

I am so happy; I had resigned myself to not being able to dive, which would have been a total bummer – especially if I was the only one out of the four of us. The problem is now resolved. I had got a copy of the dive school medical form and it was now all complete and signed off, so hopefully no problem.

The end of term comes and it an emotional time, as my year group partner, who I have worked with for the last two years, is leaving to go back home to South Africa. The good thing is he is going to house-sit for us while we are away; a win-win as far as I am concerned. I have also decided to work part time. I had put in a request to drop down to three days a week and as someone was coming back from maternity leave and also wanted to work part time, I was in luck.

I also feel the need to do this because John has changed jobs again. A good change; he has gone back to work with Ray at Rexam. He had been so unhappy in the end at ICI Paints that he had approached Rexam to see if there were any vacancies and they had him back almost straight away. This time he is based in Luton rather than Milton Keynes, but he still has to travel quite a lot. With the best will in the world, I cannot work full time at teaching, organise a house and get my children to all the places they need to be – swimming, music, scouts etc. There is a saying that part time teachers work full time and that full time teachers work all the time. I spend at least two or three evenings a week working for at least two hours a night on my planning. If John was away, this would not be possible. I have also been thinking for a while that perhaps my body is trying to tell me something.

The end of June also brings my follow-up visit with Simon Jennings. Firstly, he gives me a disk with a copy of the photos of my hip, then we get down to the nitty gritty of why I am still having consistent pain in the hip. Walking is OK, but the minute I have to lift my leg up, if sitting or lying down I get sharp pains. Sneezing or coughing also hurts quite a bit too. I know I sound like I am moaning and I don't mean to, I should be grateful that I am no longer in agony with every step I take, but it is hard to still feel like this. I hadn't expected that I would be running marathons (not that I ever had) but I would like to be able to get in and out of the car without having to use my hands to lift my right leg in and out.

He shows me the results of the post surgical x-ray and he is able to reassure me that the new joint is fine and that my pain is not directly due to this. He suggests an ultrasound scan and if necessary a cortisone injection in the tendon to relieve the pain, which will also help with diagnosing the problem.

This is arranged for the Monday after term finishes. I have the scan with the same doctor who has given me the last two injections. I chat away as normal; driving him to distraction I am sure. He comments that there is a small amount of swelling on the Illeosoas (hip flexor) tendon and that he can inject it to see if it will help with the pain. I am at this point prepared to try anything and so say yes please! The injection is painful and I get the feeling straight away that it won't make much difference. This is because the effect has been fairly instantaneous with the last two and I don't feel like this now. It can't do any harm though, so I hope that the benefit will be delayed.

The first week of the summer holidays rushes by as I get everything ready for our Australian trip of a lifetime. Lizzie is away in Brittany with Harrow Young Musicians and comes back midweek and then it is time to tidy the house and get it ready for Ron and his family to come and stay. Friday comes and the bags are packed, we take the rabbits to Maureen who looks after them for us and all is ready.

CHAPTER 28

Travel Broadens the Mind and Brings Friends Closer

Saturday morning come and we are off to the airport for the mammoth flight to Perth via Singapore. We are flying with Qantas and we get to go on one of the massive new A380 airbuses – a double decker plane, amazing. Our plan includes catching up with lots of friends and also visiting lots of key places. First stop Perth, to stay with the Woodhams, friends of John's from university. We spend each evening relaxing with them after seeing the sights of Perth and Fremantle. It is fun for the children and we fall in love with their dogs. Staying with friends is wonderful; you really get to know them in a much more meaningful way. It is not that you have known them superficially, but when you stay with someone you get a real taste of what their life is like.

Debbie and Andy are two very special people. They have three lovely boys, the oldest two are both autistic. What can I say, except that I am in awe of how they have managed their lives and how they have managed with what may, to most people, seem very adverse circumstances. Debbie is inspirational in how she deals with the two boys, who to many would be considered to have quite challenging behaviour. Andy makes the point that managing people in commerce is a complete doddle after handling the challenges that Elliott and Scott can give them. It is an enlightening experience and a real privilege to spend time with such a special family.

Again, I reflect that the human spirit is truly amazing. So many different individuals have to manage so many different difficulties that life throws at them. Mine pale into insignificance in comparison to what Debbie and Andy have had to deal with, and will have to deal with for the rest of their lives. They do so without complaint or dissention and continually battle against the prejudices that society has for the behavioural norms. I can tell that this trip is going to be very special and that staying with Andy, Debbie and the boys is going to be hard to beat.

Then to Uluru, a definite bucket list contender. Seeing Ayers Rock, as it used to be called, is something that I have wanted to do since I saw a photograph of it in *National Geographic* when I was a child. We are staying in a family room and so it is going to be very cosy. I have arranged a full itinerary for the three days we are staying here. We have a sunset dinner, where I get to see the Milky Way for the first time in my life. The morning after we arrive we get up at 5.00am to start a pre-dawn walk to see sunrise over the giant, red monolith. We have a guided 14km walk around Uluru with a Kiwi guide, who gives us the simplest version of the Aboriginal legends of both Uluru and Kata Tjuta (what used to be known as The Olgas). Now, remember it is the Australian Winter and we are smack in the middle of an exceedingly large continent. It is nearly freezing. I had told everyone to dress warmly, but they had not really listened. Despite the cold, by the time the sun comes up we are afforded some spectacular views of some of the most unusual scenery in the world, so soon forget how freezing it had been.

My hip is bearing up and although the flights are a bit uncomfortable, the walking is proving beneficial. We have another meal out under the stars that night and the following morning board a short, light aircraft flight over the rock. Marcus is desperate to become a pilot and so he is happy as a lark to be sitting in the co-pilot's seat. The whole experience is fantastic, but for me, learning about the Aboriginal culture was most fascinating. You know, western society could learn an awful lot from such a wise race of people. I am amazed to discover whilst there that you can actually walk up Uluru, or rather climb, using the chain that is fixed into the most accessible slope of the rock. The Annanu people ask that you don't climb it; this is not due to the fact that parts of Uluru are sacred, but more from the responsibility they feel for anyone who might hurt themselves on their land. Climbing is inherently risky, especially when it is hot. In fact, you are not allowed to climb after 8am during the hotter months as the iron oxide rock coating gets so hot, it will melt the soles of your shoes!

One week in and we are off to Cairns so we can learn to dive. Debbie and Andy had recommended a visit to Kuranda Skyrail and to the rainforest. When we get to our apartment in Cairns we arrange this, as we have a spare day on Monday. This was originally kept empty so that I could have my special medical, but as I am now sorted it means we have a day to be tourists rather than mess around getting medical stuff sorted. It is a fantastic day, but another very early start. That night we eat in the Balinese restaurant at the hotel/apartment block – it is the children's first experience of Indonesian food and they love it.

On Tuesday it is time to learn to dive. Dave, our instructor, picks us up bright and early and we spend the morning in the classroom and the afternoon in the pool. At lunchtime, John and the children have their medicals. Boy I am glad I had mine in England, there is no way this doctor would have passed me. They are very conservative and safety conscious. Rightly so, however, the Australian culture has become so litigious that the pendulum has swung too far, perhaps.

The morning's lessons make me realise how dangerous diving really is, and the afternoon in the pool reinforces that. The worst part for me is that I am so buoyant – remember fat is lighter than muscle – I have to have seven weights on my belt, totalling 10.5kg

I FELT A RIGHT ONE...

in all. Believe me, that is bloody heavy. I have more weights than John. Walking with the wetsuit, all the weights, the buoyancy control device (BCD), tank and air regulators means I am carrying about 18-20kg of kit in total. That is quite a strain on my new hip and my neck doesn't like the weight much either.

Once in the water the difficulty is removed and you realise that the physical difficulties on land are only brief in comparison to the most amazingly liberating time in the water. This time with the family learning do to something that I had wanted to do for over twenty years is incredibly special. 'Living for the moment' may seem an overused phrase, but it is so important. It is a real shame that it takes major life events to make us realise it, but I am so glad that I have learnt this lesson and, fortunately, not too late.

Two days in the classroom and pool and then three days out on a boat on the barrier reef itself. Wow, what can I say, it is the most amazingly beautiful place in the world. We had spent an evening at a marine biology lecture, called 'reef teach', so that whilst diving, we actually have some idea of what we are looking at. On the boat, I am beginning to find things a bit of a strain on the hip, but the crew are amazing and arrange to carry all my kit to the dive entry point and then help me take it all off before getting out of the water. I don't manage quite as many dives as the rest of the family, but I pass and qualify for my PADI open water certificate, so I am more than happy. The children are desperate to complete their adventure diver certificate and so we spend a little more money (an advance Christmas present) and they get certified to dive deeper than either John or I.

We leave Cairns and fly to Brisbane, where we have a hire car organised. We drive north 100 miles or so to the Sunshine Coast and stay in a wonderful place in the Mulloolah Valley. There we meet up with Melissa and Luke; Melissa taught at my school for six months about three years ago and it is so lovely to see them. The next day we head off on our three day drive to Sydney. We have not planned any accommodation and are just going to take things as we find them. Resting in the car is actually quite good for the kids, as the holiday has been pretty full-on so far. We drive through the Glasshouse Mountains, go to Byron Bay, into Dorrigo and then down the Waterfall Way. We stay in Coolangatta, Nambucca Heads and finally end up in the Hunter Valley. Four vineyards and the only brewery in the wine region is completed in under a day and then it is off to Sydney.

We are staying with Nic and Susie. I have known Nic for nearly forty years and it is great to spend time with good friends again. We have our first home cooked meal in Australia. From there we go to Mosman in central Sydney, right by the harbour, to stay with Rachel, my oldest friend who I have known since primary school, so about forty-five years.

For me, seeing all these friends is the highlight of the trip. Yes, seeing all the cultural and natural wonders that Australia has to offer is brilliant, but it is the people that matter the most. Friends, especially ones you have known for a long time, are very special. It seems that it does not matter how long it is since you have last seen them, you just pick up from where you left off.

Family is important as well, of course, but truly friends are the most important. I count John as my best friend and he is also my husband. I am lucky that I have a wonderful family and that I am also, through marriage, part of a fantastic family. Many of them are friends also. As I get older and more happens, friendships are even more meaningful. This whole trip has been to see and do wonderful things and to share those experiences with my husband and children, but visiting the friends is probably the most important highlight for me.

When we arrive, Rachel takes us driving around the north shore to get our bearings and then that evening we go off to have dinner at another friend's house in Hunters Hill. I met Lorraine when I was eleven and we have stayed in contact ever since. As John is flying home tomorrow we wanted to catch them before he left. I feel guilty arriving at Rachel's and then going off to see someone else, but I know she understands. Again, catching up with Lorraine and her family means the children get to spend some time with other children/young people, even if not quite the same age. I think they may be getting a little bored of John's and my company!

The next morning we make a whistle stop tour of central Sydney with John and then return home to Rachel's house to say our farewells to him. He is taking the hire car back to the airport when he goes and we will use public transport for the rest of the week. I am so sad to see him go and know that both the children and I will miss him hugely. Lizzie, Marcus and I spend another four days with Rachel, Gary, Fraser and Martha. Emily is away in Canada, but it is her birthday whilst we are there and the family Skype her to celebrate.

It is truly relaxing here. We are made to feel so at home and I can tell the children are pleased just to spend some time vegetating and watching DVDs, recovering from all the sightseeing, which of course we still do a lot more of. Sally the Labradoodle is also a big hit, especially with Marcus; he sits and cuddles her at any opportunity. I can see that I am going to get nagged constantly when we get home about getting a dog.

On Wednesday we leave for the airport to fly to the USA. I am sad to leave Rachel and although we will be in Facebook and email contact, I don't know when I will get to see her next. The time spent with her and the family has been incredibly memorable. My children have seen, at first hand, how long friendships can last and how important they are. Marcus made a comment to me that Rachel and I were both very similar and he was surprised that we actually got on so well. It makes me reflect on what makes friendships last: shared values and beliefs. For Rachel and me, in the particular, the fact that we are also both a little manic, highly organised, extrovert and care passionately about family and friends is something to be proud of!

The final leg of our amazing trip now unfolds, with a ridiculously long flight to LA and then a quick change down to San

Fransisco. We cross the International Date Line and seem to get Wednesday all over again. More wonderful friends await us here. This time another friend that Rachel and I were at primary school with, Rowena, is our host. I haven't seen Rowena since I was eleven, but we reconnected through Rachel on Facebook. To say I am excited is the understatement of the year. Rowena has arranged for her husband Alan to collect us and he is duly waiting with a sign with our names on. It is a little unnerving to be hosted so wonderfully by someone you have never met before, but Alan is the perfect host and drives us down to where they live in San Jose.

Sleep deprivation is starting to take effect, but the children are really excited. We arrive at the house and I get to be reunited with Rowena. We had been in email contact before we left and Rowena has also pre-read a copy of this book for me. We are only staying with her for one night and we cram in lots.

The key thing the children want to do in the US is clothes shop, because it is so much cheaper than in the UK. Rowena gets out the Porsche to take us to the mall. The children cannot keep the smile off their faces and as I sit and write this I am beaming as well. Two hours of shopping and I am ready to drop, then back for a lovely barbecue and the children get to have a swim. Rowena's lovely springer spaniels are lots of fun too.

In the morning more shopping, a lovely lunch at Santana Row and then Rowena drives us to Palo Alto to stay with Jackie Cook. Jackie and I used to work together at 3, in Maidenhead. Jackie, Tony and their four boys moved to the US about four years ago and I haven't seen her since then. Another dog for my children to admire and more children to play with. All a little younger, but different company than just me.

We are staying with them for two nights and Tony is kindly driving us into San Francisco for our Alcatraz tour. A whole day walking up and down very big hills is exhausting then we walk to Tony's office and he brings us home. On our last morning Tony is amazing and takes his four children and Lizzie and Marcus to a theme park, so that Jackie and I can have a quiet morning catching up and just spending time together. We go to downtown Palo Alto, have coffee and do last bits of shopping for me, which includes 6kg of peanut butter M&Ms!

Again I appreciate the time spent with people that I love and care about. When friends move abroad it is a huge effort for them to leave all their family and circle of friends at home. I am really appreciating more and more how happy they are to have visitors (if not they have done ever such a good job hiding it!) It keeps the friendships alive, you see how they are living and so in the future when they talk about their time in these places you know and understand more about their experiences. It therefore takes the friendships to a new place. You have a better understanding of how they live their lives according to the similarities and differences to your own. Of course visiting friends also means that you get to see places you might not have otherwise. It cements relationships, gives you a mental map of their situation and they appreciate the effort you have made to visit them. It brings your friendship up to date in a meaningful way.

Lizzie and Marcus have said to me that they feel like they live in a bed and breakfast. We have a spare bedroom in our loft-conversion. It is very regularly used by friends and family who come to visit from different parts of this country and all over the world. Lizzie also says that once you are my friend, you are always my friend and that you are very unlikely to escape! To a certain extent that is true; over the last couple of years I have learnt that I really do need people. I feed off the energy created when people get together, so keeping a room always at the ready for any friends who want to come and stay is just a natural extension of that. These same friends whether near or far are the ones who keep you going, whose kind words support you when you are down, whose thoughts and prayers provide a wall of positive energy which cocoons you from any negativity that may try to creep in. Friends are a comfort blanket, a force field, a safety net, an essential oil for your soul. Life without friends is like what I imagine drowning would be like. Not something that I want to imagine at all, really.

So, our trip which has reunited us with seven different friends and their families has been truly wonderful, but it now comes to an end. We make the flight home and John collects us from the airport. An overnighter again with no sleep for me and little for the children means that when we get home Marcus actually falls asleep with his head in his hands lying on the floor. He says that evening, that although it was brilliant, he never wants to go on a holiday like that again as it was so tiring. Wow, I have managed to exhaust my ever ready, bunny style teenage son!

CHAPTER 29

Coming of Age

With all the health issues over the last three years, I had decided to go part time and was lucky enough to be able to do so. John will be doing more travelling again and I have decided that working full time, running a house, getting two children to all the activities and a husband away a fair bit, is not conducive to a stress-free life.

One of the things that having cancer has taught me is that reducing the stress in your life is important. I do appreciate that I am lucky enough to be able to work part time, however with such a drastic cut in my salary a few things will need to change. I let my cleaner go before the holidays started and now I invest in a steamer to make ironing a lot easier and so I don't send it out any more. The recession is really starting to bite and we also need to think about tightening our belt. We get a clothes line in the garden, as I actually have time to hang out washing (weather dependent of course!)

I am teaching Wednesday, Thursday and Friday, but I go in for staff training on a Monday afternoon after school. I do find myself needing to do a little overtime, but all in all I am really enjoying not having to work in the evenings. Any extra marking or school work I need to do, I do on my days off so that I can actually spend time with the family in the evenings, rather than being closeted in the study three nights a week planning my lessons. The stress is definitely less.

This is Lizzie's GCSE year and Marcus will also be choosing his options. It makes me think that if both my children want to go off to University or join the Air Force (which is Marcus' current career choice), then I will only have my children at home with me for another four years. Only four years; another good reason to have more time to spend with them.

More and more I have been thinking about what I want to do with the rest of my life. Do I want to climb the ladder in the teaching profession? Do I want the stress that would come with that? I don't know, is the answer. I do know that I love teaching and being in the classroom, so for the moment I am going to enjoy that and enjoy my life with my family. Who knows what is round the corner? I really appreciate how lucky I am and just want to enjoy being.

Now Autumn is here, it is time to think about celebrating my big birthday. I cannot believe that I am about to turn fifty. Mentally, I feel like I am in my thirties, my body of course tells me different. However, I cannot let this major milestone in my life pass by without a celebration. Of course it turns into a big one and 150 people later, I have a fantastic birthday bash. Friends come from near and far and my house is not just a bed and breakfast, but a fully fledged hotel. Friends from France, Dubai and Wales are booked in. Amazingly Chris, from Arizona turns up as a surprise at the party and so he joins the throng with a mattress on the lounge floor with Hunty. We follow up by having a breakfast party for about twenty who had stayed over locally the next morning.

I had asked specifically for no presents, but that if people felt they wanted to give then a donation to St Luke's would be great. In the end when I count it all up, people have given over £1,500. I am overwhelmed and so grateful. It is hard to decide how to mark such an occasion, but, for me I feel it is important to celebrate, because indeed I have so much to celebrate. How often in life to do we get the opportunity to get all our friends and family together? Of course, some people can't come, but they are definitely there in spirit.

CHAPTER 30

A New Nipple and a Proper Tattoo

Once the entire birthday hullabaloo is over, it is time to think of the final stages of rebuilding my body. I arrange an appointment with Adam Searle to talk about nipple reconstruction. John comes with me as usual; for me it is really important that he is part of the process. He is able to keep track of my frame of mind and also understand the implications of all the decisions I am making about any treatments that I choose to have. Although I am making the decisions for me, they do ultimately affect him as well.

Adam has a look at his handiwork to see how it has settled after a year. I update him on the hip replacement and he just looks at me with a smile and makes some comment about me being amazing. A lovely thing to say, even though I don't think I am.

Now to update you on what my chest actually looks like. My new right breast, nipple-less, sits higher than the left one and has a scar right across it and the other scar is tucked underneath where the breast drops down. My left one is slightly lower and still a little bigger than my reconstructed one, even after two reductions. However, when I wear a bra, which is how most people see me, you wouldn't really notice the difference. Some women have naturally different sized breasts anyway and most women are not symmetrical either, so I am totally delighted. I definitely have a better figure and now the hip problem is solved, I have even lost a little weight.

Adam is happy to consider the nipple reconstruction and explains again how he would do it. We talk about how long the recovery would be and also about the tattooing of the areola to complete the process. I decided that early in the New Year would be a good time to get it done.

Many women don't bother with this final stage and some women just decide to get the nipple tattooed on. However, having gone through three significant operations to get here, one more small procedure is nothing.

So in March 2012, three years and four months after my original mastectomy, I have my final surgical procedure to complete my reconstruction and half an hour later I have a new nipple. I have to keep a doughnut of sponge around it until all the stitches are out, so that my lovely new nipple doesn't get flattened whilst it is healing.

I post an update on Facebook that day. I have to include it here as so many of the comments had me in hysterics!

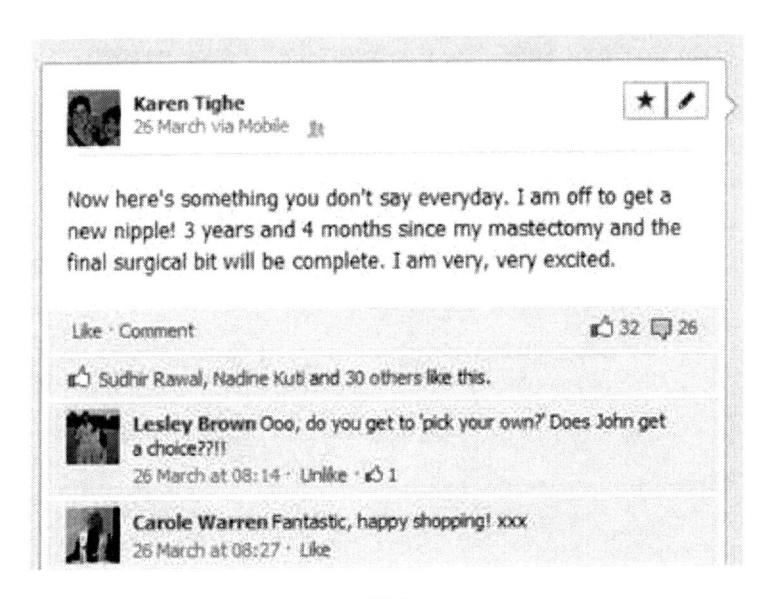

Karen Tighe
26 March via Mobile

Now here's something you don't say everyday. I am off to get a new nipple! 3 years and 4 months since my mastectomy and the final surgical bit will be complete. I am very, very excited.

Like · Comment   32   26

Sudhir Rawal, Nadine Kuti and 30 others like this.

Lesley Brown Ooo, do you get to 'pick your own?' Does John get a choice??!!
26 March at 08:14 · Unlike · 1

Carole Warren Fantastic, happy shopping! xxx
26 March at 08:27 · Like

I FELT A RIGHT ONE...

Sharla Bloxham Over 3 years ago? No way!
26 March at 08:32 · Like

Geri Ellis Now that is the most unusual status I have ever read on fb. Needed to reread it a few times. Good luck
26 March at 08:56 · Like

Fizah Durrani Samar Easy Karen, your excitement may now be very noticeable with the new nipple in place!!! Good luck xx
26 March at 12:43 · Like

Rowena Cherry Nipple congrats :) xxx
26 March at 14:27 · Like · 👍 1

Zoe Tighe Congratulations. Happy nipple day!
26 March at 14:48 · Like

Cameron Murray Tattooed nipple?
26 March at 15:17 · Like

Karen Tighe Not yet. Need to wait for 6 weeks or so for that. I have always wanted a tattoo. I am wondering if I should ask for a flower or something!!
26 March at 15:26 · Like · 👍 3

Jon Cobb Is it high-tech with different spray options - jet, super-soaker, fine mist etc?
26 March at 17:30 · Unlike · 👍 1

Rose Warren voila....http://www.google.co.uk/imgres?um=1&hl=en&client=firefox-a&rls=org.mozilla%3Aen-GB%3Aofficial&biw=1252&bih=595&tbm=isch&tbnid=Spm HyItcUZIWnM%3A&imgrefurl=http%3A%2F%2Fbyebyehooters. blogspot.com%2F2010%2F06%2Ffloral-tattoo-or-normal-n ipples.html&docid=Trk3-kg86n7aAM&imgurl=http%3A%2F%2 F1.bp.blogspot.com%2F_yh3nXUdS3Fo%2FTAz5pKiy_6I%2FAA AAAAAAB2s%2FxiXyRLtVztc%2Fs1600%2Funtitled.bmp&w=350 8h=1918&ei=x6hwT7OlGcG_0QWc 4cGNAg&zoom=1&iact=hc&vpx= 403&vpy=167&dur=210&hovh=1 52&hovw=280&tx=187&ty=68&sig=10517202774382854028989 age=1&tbnh=98&tbnw=179&start=0&ndsp=18&ved=1t% 3A429%2Cr%3A2%2Cs%3A0

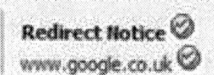

Redirect Notice
www.google.co.uk

26 March at 18:36 · Unlike · 👍 3 · Remove preview

Well worth looking at this link!

A New Nipple and a Proper Tattoo

Rowena Cherry Wow pretty! The flowery tatt nipps....
26 March at 18:40 · Like

Cameron Murray You know everyone; young and old will be asking you to flash your boobs at them from now on! :)
26 March at 18:43 · Like

Zoe Tighe Cameron....... I thought the same thing!!!!
26 March at 18:59 · Like

Freddie Shirley How on earth do you select - is there like a nipple display counter? Do they do BOGOF?
26 March at 19:03 · Unlike · 1

Freddie Shirley Mike has just asked if you can have it pre-pierced?
26 March at 19:03 · Like · 1

Rowena Cherry Of course we'll all wanna see!!!!
26 March at 19:37 · Like · 1

Karen Tighe Cam after my main reconstruction op I got them out at a dinner party. Needless to say I had had a glass of sparkly stuff or two!! I think I may have embarrassed a couple of people.
26 March at 19:51 · Like · 2

Karen Tighe Freddie, Lizzie had told me to ask Adam, my plastic surgeon (doesn't that sound posh) if I could have one with flashing lights. He said no, but I wasn't the first person to ask!!
26 March at 19:58 · Like · 3

Gill Ross Is that cherry picking? Or pick your own or if its tartan would it be the Edinburgh Tatoo...enough already!
26 March at 20:58 · Unlike · 1

Julie Scott Good luck x
26 March at 22:32 · Like

Cameron Murray ...isnt it lovely that we can all now joke about what was once a truly scary subject for you. BTW you have to post a fb picture of the "nips" when you get them!
26 March at 22:42 · Like

Karen Tighe Mmmm. I am not sure I am that brave :-). You know Cam, I have been so lucky all the way through this and I now have a better figure than before. So every cloud has a silver lining.
26 March at 22:54 · Like · 1

Wendy Barber Being one of the people at the dinner party where you exposed yourself Karen we are hoping for a repeat performance with the new nipples!! Tim still hasn't recovered!
27 March at 20:28 · Like · 1

I FELT A RIGHT ONE...

> **Renee Smoyer Weissend** congrats on finishing up the process.
> 28 March at 19:56 · Like
>
> **Lesley Brown** How about the HSMCC crest?
> 30 March at 21:48 · Like

I must say, that I am a great Facebook fan and this is an example of why I think so.

Anyway, I visit once a week for the next three weeks to have the stitches removed. By the end of this I have a lovely nipple which, when naked, sits slightly higher than my left one, but whilst wearing a bra gives just enough lift to make me more symmetrical, especially in tight fitting clothing. Six week later at the beginning of May I return for the first of my nipple tattooing sessions! Adam had explained that it would be best to tattoo both nipples so that they matched better. I had assumed I would get an anaesthetic on the left one, knowing that the new one has no feeling so wouldn't matter anyway.

Well I was wrong and I will prepare for my next session by going to Boots and getting some of that numbing cream they put on children's arms before having an injection! Nipples are quite sensitive and to start with it was alright, but by the end it really was quite sore. Another great thing that Shelley the tattooist did was try to cover up the bright blue radiotherapy dot in the middle of my chest. This is taking a little longer to heal so we will wait and see what happens.

Even after this first round the effect is truly amazing. Whilst walking round the bathroom after a shower or bath, when I catch a glimpse of myself in the mirror I look normal again. Yes, there is scarring on both the breasts, but as this fades they are just white lines that pale into the background. My new nipple is like the cherry on the cake, almost literally, but definitely metaphorically.

The other day when I was relaxing in the bath, John was sitting chatting to me and I could see him looking at my chest. "That is unbelievable," he said "you would never know it was not real. These surgeons are so clever aren't they?"

I think it helps him forget too and for that I am very glad.

Summer half term comes and it is time for the final finishing touches; the last tattoo. I use the cream to numb the skin on the left nipple and head off to London again. Shelley completes the process and it is home again. It takes about three weeks for all the skin to recover and finally, I am complete.

Wow. What a journey, what an experience.

CHAPTER 31

Life is a Journey

As my story draws to a close, I start to reread all that I have written and realise that this book starts with us visiting friends and ends talking about friends; starts with us watching one Olympics and ends with me in full preparation to volunteer for the London 2012 Olympics; starts with me discovering I am sick and ends with the completion of me being rebuilt. Life is a journey, a journey that has pattern and meaning to it. Two important parts of my life are friends and being active, the part about getting sick is just a small blip in an otherwise wonderful journey.

Don't I wish that when I was a child I had the wisdom I have now, well maybe not wisdom, but knowledge. Having said that, I don't really regret anything. I don't mean at the end of this book to go all philosophical on you or anything, but these issues certainly do make you think. Thinking is a good thing; thinking makes you realise the value of what you have.

Life is wonderful and is to be enjoyed. Since having cancer I can honestly say that I truly do appreciate *everything* more. I hope that I am less judgemental now. You never know what is going on in someone else's mind, or why; you never know what they might be going through and why. No one has the right to judge. Not everyone is the same and just because I might be extrovert and out there, others are not and so I cannot impose my way on them. I must just accept them for what they are; I don't have to like it, I just have to accept it.

Being positive is in my nature, it is at my very core, but experiencing such a serious life event has made me even more so. Being negative brings you down and others with you. We all have a responsibility to be the best person we can be, no matter what our circumstances. The saying that I seem to hear so often now, 'life is not a rehearsal' takes on greater meaning. We have to live with what we have done; we have to accept that we cannot change the past. A life of 'what-ifs' is not a life at all.

As I finally complete this book, the Olympics has just finished and the Paralympics is soon to start. What an experience: I was working as a team leader looking after journalists in the press tribune for Table Tennis at the Excel 1 Arena. It was manic, tiring, exhilarating, fun and above all a worthwhile way to spend some time. I felt hugely privileged to watch world class sport. Not one that I had much experience of before, but an incredibly skilled and fascinating one nevertheless. I met many interesting people, journalists and officials from all over the world, all of whom were amazingly positive about London. I was chosen to meet David Cameron when he visited the Excel Centre specifically to meet some volunteers. I also saw Bill Gates sit in front of our our Tribune and many international athletes cheering on their own country. I made new friends and discovered links with many old ones. It seems to me the teaching and sports world is quite small. I would describe the experience as a privilege and I am so glad that I was able to be part of something so special.

Mostly I am thankful, thankful for my wonderful husband. I forget sometimes how he might worry and I am reminded that if you are married or have a partner, the journey through any serious disease, physical or mental health problem is one that is shared. I think the balance is a little uneven, to be honest; the burden of worry for the partner can be more than for the patient sometimes, particularly with cancer. Being positive is therefore even more important, because of the impact it has on the people around you and especially those that are closest. I am thankful also for my children. The ages that they were and are at as I have gone through this has meant that I have worried a lot about their thoughts and feelings. Lizzie has now sat her GCSEs (results next week) and is aiming for medical school, she jokes that I have been a great introduction to the field. Marcus is a typical teenage boy, but loving and caring and I could not be prouder of them both.

Is it just because I am getting older that I now know more people who have serious illnesses? Is it because as one ages, you get to know more people, so there is an increase in the number of friends, so an increased likelihood that you will know someone who has had something significant happen to them? Over the last year good friends have had much more serious cancers than me, accidents have happened and people have died.

Earlier this year, a friend's daughter had an accident whilst snowboarding and is now quadriplegic. This has put my whole situation into perspective. Yes, I got cancer fairly young (forty-six), but my friend's daughter is twenty-two and will be confined to a wheelchair for the rest of her life. (My biggest hope and prayer is that medical science will advance so that this situation is not permanent for her.) With very limited movement and all that being quadriplegic entails, it makes me realise that life is a gift and one we must not take for granted. The strength, courage and positivity are a credit to my friend, her injured daughter and their family. I aspire to be as amazing and will try never to complain about not being able to do anything in life that I want to ever again. I am not sure I will achieve that, but I am really going to try.

The treatment for breast cancer is progressing and many of the women I meet in the breast care group are now having their chemotherapy in advance of their surgery. This may allow them to have less tissue removed and therefore need less reconstruction afterwards. For my type of cancer, that was not an option. Some of the ladies have had recurrences, in fact some have had the cancer come back two or three times. You have to be realistic; I have taken as much control over my life and the things that can have an impact on getting cancer as I feel I can, without actually causing myself stress. Whatever is going to happen will happen and I will deal with any recurrence if it comes along. I am certainly not going to sit around and worry that it will. I intend to live my life as if the cancer is not coming back and I intend to live it as fully as possible. No matter what happens in the future, I can have no regrets and I will leave none for those around me to deal with.

Acknowledgments

First and foremost I would like to thank all of the medical staff at the Clementine Churchil Hospital, especially Michael Burke, David Fermont, Cleo and Elaine. Also, Adam Searle and his team at his consulting rooms and at the Royal Marsden Hospital.

Jon Cobb, for inspiring this book; he really needs to publish one himself as his story is both moving and incredibly funny.

All my tremendous friends and colleagues for their support, love, time, comfort and generosity.

The children I have taught and who have had to put up with me during this process.

Jean Gaffin, for helping with the very first edit, Rowena Cherry, Lisa Allera, Colleen Wood and Sarah Darnell who have helped and advised, by proof reading and giving me feedback.

Last but not least, my family, most especially my amazing husband, without whom I would be lost. His sense of humour and the fact that he can make me laugh at anything is a wonderful gift. Lizzie and Marcus are truly a blessing, they love life and smile so much that spending time with them is always a pleasure.

Thanks to Lizzie for the Front cover picture and to John, Lizzie and Marcus for all the other photos included here.